U0382102

大变局下的
博弈与合作

GAME AND COOPERATION

UNDER PROFOUND CHANGES

王灵桂　**主编**

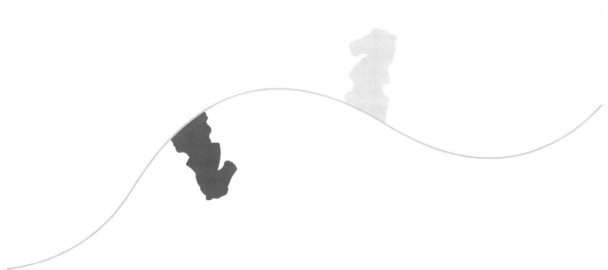

中国社会科学出版社

图书在版编目（CIP）数据

大变局下的博弈与合作/王灵桂主编．—北京：中国社会科学出版社，
2021.10

ISBN 978 - 7 - 5203 - 8034 - 8

Ⅰ.①大… Ⅱ.①王… Ⅲ.①新型冠状病毒肺炎—疫情管理—
世界—文集 Ⅳ.①R563.1 - 53

中国版本图书馆 CIP 数据核字（2021）第 193417 号

出 版 人	赵剑英
责任编辑	喻 苗
责任校对	闫 萃
责任印制	王 超

出 版	中国社会科学出版社
社 址	北京鼓楼西大街甲 158 号
邮 编	100720
网 址	http://www.csspw.cn
发 行 部	010 - 84083685
门 市 部	010 - 84029450
经 销	新华书店及其他书店

印 刷	北京明恒达印务有限公司
装 订	廊坊市广阳区广增装订厂
版 次	2021 年 10 月第 1 版
印 次	2021 年 10 月第 1 次印刷

开 本	710×1000 1/16
印 张	21.25
字 数	328 千字
定 价	118.00 元

目　　录

人类命运共同体

全球化前景

国际秩序

大国关系

公共安全

中国角色

Contents

A Community of Shared Future for Mankind

International Order

Great Power Relations

Public Security

China's Role

序　言

　　新冠肺炎疫情是一场波及全球的重大公共卫生灾难。面对这场关乎生死存亡的抗疫斗争，世界各国选择了不同的符合自身国情的抗疫方式。同时，各国普遍认识到：我们同处一个地球，同处一个世界，共同面对同一场灾难，虽然技术性的应对和处理手法不同，但是大家普遍都认识到，在灾难面前，没有一个国家和地区能够独善其身，能够超然于疫情之外。只有站在整个人类命运未来的高度，搁置争端争议、加强协作协调、互相支持帮助，才能最终战胜灾难，渡过波劫。疫情在中国暴发时，世界各国给中国人民巨大的物质和道义支持。在中国疫情得到基本控制后，中国政府投桃报李，迅速向相关国家（地区）和国际组织捐赠物资、派遣专家、分享数据、交流经验。疫情无情，人间有爱，中国人民和全球人民共同谱写了彰显人类命运共同体的抗疫新篇章。中国人民铭记着国际社会的滴水之恩，世界各国也感受了中国人民的无私温暖。"亚当子孙皆兄弟"这句古语，反映了构建人类命运共同体的真实心声。

　　世界各国在抗击疫情的斗争中，集体唤醒和强化了人类共同命运意识。科学家有国界，但是科学没有国界，我们看到全球医药卫生工作者和科技工作者携手合作、共享数据和信息：中国科学家将病毒基因组排序迅速与世界各国分享、不同国家科技工作者共同研制攻克病毒的药物、共同加紧研制疫苗。人民有国界，但是互相支持和关心的道德观跨越了国界，我们看到世界各国守望相助，互赠抗疫物资，有的国家把自己最后的库存抗疫物资毫无保留地捐赠出来。这次抗疫经历，说明在疫情这个人类共同敌人面前，人类命运共同体的理念，决不是简单的口号，也不是可有可无、无足轻重的理念，而是一种事关整个人类福祉的伟大理念，是人类追求美好生活的必由之路和鲜活实践平台。

从一定意义上说，这次疫情将彻底改变人类的许多理念。面对迅速蔓延的无情疫情，各国普遍认识到，唯有以保护人类未来和人民福祉为出发点，走团结合作的命运共同体之路，才是制服新型冠状病毒肺炎的唯一正确选择。2020 年 3 月 26 日召开的 G20 领导人应对新冠病毒肺炎特别峰会，就是这个共识的里程碑式象征。第 73 届世卫组织大会的召开，也标志着国际社会开始真正面对并讨论人类社会面临的共同威胁，国际社会开启了摒弃分歧、团结协作的新范式，全球治理进入了新版本时代，中国倡导的人类命运共同体理念开始进入国际操作层面。疫情已经催生了以人类命运共同体为骨干理念的新国际价值观，实现这种理念的原则就是共商共建共享和合作共赢。

人类命运共同体理念代表着人类的进步。在以往的历次人类浩劫中，世界各国大都采取了逆来顺受、听天由命的做法。但是，此次疫情暴发在全球化已经高度发达的今天，人类事实上已经形成了空前紧密的命运共同体关系。面对全人类的共同敌人，世界各国团结起来战胜病毒的可能性已成现实，各国寻求合作抗疫也成为必然政策选项。这是人类历史上以命运共同体意识共克时艰、共抗风险的开端，标志着人类共同价值观的巨大飞跃和进步。正如习近平主席在 G20 特别峰会上强调指出的："只要我们同舟共济、守望相助，就一定能够彻底战胜疫情，迎来人类发展更加美好的明天。"全球 190 多个国家和地区、70 多亿人口，因何而紧密相连？未来又将走向何方？基于对历史和现实的深入思考，中国领导人给出了中国答案。从 2013 年年初到 2018 年年中，习近平主席在近 70 个不同的重大国内国际场合，深刻阐述了命运共同体这个宏大课题，展现了中国领导人面向未来的长远眼光、博大胸襟和历史担当。习近平主席提出，"中国的方案是：构建人类命运共同体，实现共赢共享"，"只要怀有真诚的愿望，秉持足够善意，展现政治智慧，再大的冲突都能化解，再厚的坚冰都能打破"，大道至简，实干为要，"邻居出了问题，不能光想着扎好自家篱笆，而应该去帮一把"。在这次伟大的抗疫斗争中，中国人民已经走出了坚实的一步。在这场伟大的斗争中，那些逆潮流而动者，应反思并回到正确的人类发展道路上来，共筑人类新共同价值观的基础。

王灵桂

中国社会科学院副院长、

中国社会科学院国家高端智库副理事长、研究员

2021 年 6 月 30 日

Introduction

The COVID-19 outbreak, defined by the World Health Organization as a "pandemic", is a major public health calamity in human history that spreads across the world. At present, countries all over the world have been seriously affected, and hundreds of thousands of lives have been claimed.

In the face of this battle that concerns the survival of mankind, countries all over the world have adopted different anti-epidemic measures based on their domestic conditions. Within this context, a face mask, however, has been assigned a significant political meaning. Wearing it or not has become a sign of people's political stance. It was not until the prime minister of an EU country was moved to the ICU that the political odor of the face mask began to fade away. By July 4 2020, although some people still insisted on not wearing face masks, the media began to portray them as being reckless, instead of a sign of "political correctness".

In the eyes of some Western politicians, the fight against COVID-19 could be just a string of tedious figures or a direct or indirect way to serve a certain political agenda. But it is more likely a proof of their inability to effectively organize and mobilize society and national resources to protect the life and health of citizens. That's why there has been a heated debate over the response to this life-and-death battle. A representative voice, "herd immunity", was very much talked about and supported. The spread of the coronavirus around the world is posing a threat to more and more lives. The idea of "putting people and their life and livelihood first" advocated by the Chinese government is awakening the conscience of mankind.

On June 18, 2020, in his keynote speech entitled Defeating COVID-19 with Solidarity and Cooperation at the Extraordinary China-Africa Summit on Solidarity Against COVID-19, Chinese President Xi Jinping pointed out, "COVID-19 is still affecting many parts of the world. Both China and Africa face the formidable task of combating the virus while stabilizing the economy and protecting people's livelihoods. We must always put our people and their lives front and center. We must mobilize the necessary resources, stick together in collaboration, and do whatever it takes to protect people's lives and health and minimize the fallout of COVID-19. " This is the first time that the convincing principle of putting people and their life and livelihood first has been put forward. In an interview with *Guangming Daily* on June 30, Professor Cai Fang of the Chinese Academy of Social Sciences talked of this principle, "We will never adopt the Western method of 'herd immunity' because every life is worth saving" . In an exclusive interview with *Changjiang Daily*, he further explained, "We always put people and their life first and do not take statistical risks like 'herd immunity' . Some Western countries resort to " the law of large numbers" , trying to flatten the COVID-19 curves. It seems to be a scientific and feasible measure from a statistical point of view. However, it is not acceptable according to the people-centered principle, because every percentage point of infection rate will affect health and life and every percentage of unemployment will affect livelihood. This principle, if applied to the resumption of work and economic activities, is to formulate macroeconomic policies with people and livelihood at the core.

At present, "putting people and their life and livelihood first" is becoming the mainstream anti-pandemic principle. Because, the rampant coronavirus has made the world aware that as residents of the same earth and the same world, we are faced with the same disaster. Although our response may vary, no country, region, or individual can stay safe from the pandemic. The only way to overcome COVID-19 is to bear in mind the shared future of mankind, put aside disputes, strengthen cooperation and coordination, and support each other. After the Extraordinary China-Africa Summit on Solidarity Against COVID-19, most countries all over the world believed that President Xi's support for international cooperation and multilateralism and appeal to the world to overcome difficulties together boosted the world's confidence in defeating the pandemic as soon as possible. Ronnie Lins, director of the China-Brazil Center for Research and Business, commented: "Against the backdrop of COVID-19, multilateralism has increasingly become the best way for the common development of mankind. Only with solidarity and cooperation can we defeat the coronavirus and recover the economy. " Ignacio Martinez of the National Autonomous University of Mexico commented: "President Xi Jinping's speech highlights the importance of fighting COVID-19 as one, which fully demonstrates China's attitude towards the global public health crisis. China and Africa uniting in fighting the pandemic embodies the concept of promoting the construction of a Community with a Shared Future for Mankind. "

When the coronavirus broke out, people from all over the world provided the Chinese people with tremendous material and moral support. After the coronavirus was basically under control, the Chinese government repaid their kindness by swiftly donating supplies, sending experts, sharing data, and exchanging experience. In the face of a merciless pandemic, the Chinese people and the people of the world have written a new chapter in the battle that demonstrates the Community with a Shared Future for Mankind. The Chinese people remember the kindness of the international community, and countries worldwide also sense the selflessness of the Chinese people. "The sons of Adam are limbs of each other, having been created of one essence". The saying reflects the true aspiration of building a Community with a Shared Future for Mankind.

The battle against COVID-19 has awakened and strengthened the awareness of a shared future for mankind among all countries. Science knows no national boundaries. We see that medical and health workers and scientists all over the world work together to share data and information. For instance, Chinese scientists quickly share viral genomes with other countries, and scientists from different countries speed up the development of medicine and vaccines. Moral support also goes beyond national boundaries. We see that various countries offer each other medical supplies, and some even donate the last stock of their supplies without reservation. This battle shows that in the face of COVID-19, the common enemy of humans, the concept of a Community with a Shared Future for Mankind is by no means a simple slogan or a dispensable and insignificant notion. Rather, it is a great concept concerning the well-being of mankind, the only way and a vivid platform for mankind to pursue a better life.

In a sense, the pandemic will transform many of our ideas. The rapid spread of the COVID-19 pandemic has made the world realize that only by putting the future of mankind and people's wellbeing first and building a Community with a Shared Future for Mankind featured by solidarity and cooperation that we can contain the virus. The convening of the Extraordinary China-Africa Summit on Solidarity Against COVID-19 and the previous G20 Extraordinary Leaders' Summit on COVID-19 held on March 26 are milestone symbols of this consensus. The convening of the 73rd World Health Assembly demonstrates that the international community has begun to truly face and discuss the common threats faced by human society. As the international community has started a new paradigm that puts aside differences and emphasizes solidarity and cooperation, global governance has ushered in a new era, and the concept of a Community with a Shared Future for Mankind has been put into operation worldwide. Because of COVID-19, new international values with the Community concept at the core have been formed. To turn this concept into reality, we must adhere to the principle of achieving shared growth through discussion and collaboration and win-win cooperation.

The concept of a Community with a Shared Future for Mankind represents the progress of mankind. In previous calamities, most countries could do nothing but resign themselves to their fate. However, with a high level of globalization, today's world has become an unprecedented close community with a shared future. As it is realistic for the world to act as one to defeat the virus, cooperation should become the best policy option for all countries. This will be a great moment that humans have ever surmounted difficulties with the awareness that the world is a community with a shared future. It marks significant progress in common values. As President Xi Jinping emphasized at the G20 special summit, But through solidarity and mutual assistance, we will prevail over this outbreak and we all will embrace a brighter future for mankind.

Why are we, more than 7 billion people in over 190 countries and regions, closely connected? What does the future hold? Pondering on both history and reality, Chinese leaders have provided the Chinese answers. From the beginning of 2013 to mid-2018, President Xi Jinping had expounded the Community with a Shared Future for Mankind on nearly 70 different domestic and international occasions, displaying his long-term vision, broad mind, and historical responsibility. President Xi said, "China stands for building a community of shared future for mankind and achieving inclusive and win-win development. When we have sincerity wish, goodwill, and political wisdom, no conflict is too big to settle and no ice is too thick to break. Great visions can be realized only through actions. When neighbors are in trouble, instead of tighening his own fences, one should extend a helping hand to them."

The world we live in today has been undergoing tremendous changes that are unseen in a century. The "black swan" pandemic has made changes even more complicated. In this historic battle, the Chinese people have taken a solid step forward. The splendid outcome of the battle has impressed the entire world and proved once again the Chinese government's ruling principle of serving the people wholeheartedly. In the face of this great life-and-death fight against COVID-19, those who go against the mainstream must wake up as soon as possible and return to the correct development path as soon as possible, so that the significance of face masks will be restored.

As I am writing this article, by 6: 44 pm on July 5, confirmed cases have reached 4398369 outside China, including 528955 deaths, with a rapid increase in new cases. Given such a grim situation, people all over the world should unite to oppose the politicization and the labeling of COVID-19, racial discrimination, and ideological prejudice, safeguard the global governance system with the United Nations at the core and support the World Health Organization to make greater contributions to the global fight against the pandemic. We must firmly defend international fairness and justice and moral conscience while consolidating the foundation for new common values of mankind under the guidance of the concept of building a Community with a Shared Future for Mankind.

Hereby the preamble.

Wang Linggui
Senior Research Fellow, Vice President of CASS,
Vice Chairman of Board of Directors, National Top Think
Tank Council, Chinese Academy of Social Sciences
June 30, 2021

生命至上、民生至上

蔡　昉[*]

2020 年，对中国和世界来说，都是一个特殊重要的年份。按照党的十九大部署，这一年将宣告全面建成小康社会宏伟目标的实现，具有标志性的经济社会发展指标——国内生产总值（GDP）和城乡居民收入将在 2010 年基础上分别翻一番，农村贫困人口按现行标准实现全部脱贫。然而，2020 年春节前后新冠肺炎疫情暴发始料未及地严重干扰了正常的社会经济活动，对完成全年经济社会发展目标带来严峻的挑战。全球大流行（世界卫生组织定义的疾病传播最高级别）几乎蔓延到所有国家和地区，世界主要经济体皆遭受疫情的严重冲击，进而分别因主动隔离产生的经济活动萎缩，或因主动调整或恐慌引起市场震荡，使世界经济迅速进入衰退状态。

2020 年，我们见证了什么是生命至上、民生至上的执政理念。面对疫情，不同国家采取不同的做法。西方一些国家搞平滑曲线的做法，是着眼于"大数定律"。单纯从统计学意义上看，这似乎是科学的、可行的。但是，因为每例感染者，事关的都是健康和生命，因此真正秉持生命至上、民生至上理念的执政者，是难以也不会接受"大数定律"的。

中国抗击疫情和复苏经济则遵循生命至上、民生至上的原则。我们不搞"群体免疫"那样的统计冒险。我们坚持了在每一个阶段上必要的防控措施，在较短的时间里争取到一个倒 V 字形的流行病学曲线。我们的工作步骤尊重流行病学曲线的规律，同时也以自己的努力

* 蔡昉，中国社会科学院国家高端智库首席专家、学部委员。

改变了这个曲线。

一　生命至上：中国抗击疫情的根本性原则

新型冠状病毒对生命和健康的伤害固然对所有人"一视同仁"，但是，在富裕国家和贫穷国家之间，在不同收入水平的群体之间，基本健康状态存在巨大差异，对于获得免疫、治疗、康复机会的可得性，以及受疫情经济冲击的程度和承受力都是不尽相同的。诺贝尔经济学奖获得者安格斯·迪顿在回顾疫情大流行和人类抗击历史时指出，预防和治疗流行性传染病的技术，通常是按照社会等级序列自上而下逐级传递的。因此，对这位揭示美国"绝望而死"现象的经济学家来说，在病毒面前，并非人人生而平等。

诚然，在现代社会，医疗技术的普惠性和可得性大大提高，而且，面对新型冠状病毒，无论是发达国家的亿万富翁和政要精英，还是发展中国家挣扎在贫困线上的非正规就业者，确有同样多的机会受到感染，受到感染后都会付出健康甚至生命的代价。然而，避免感染是否有选择的机会、患病后能够获得怎样的救治、疫苗一旦面世能否及时受益，特别是受疫情冲击的影响性质和程度如何，却毋庸置疑地存在着国家之间和社会人群之间的巨大差异。美国许多数据显示，非洲裔和拉丁美洲裔美国人感染新冠病毒肺炎后死亡率数倍于白种人，这些事实便是大流行面前并非人人平等这一假说的最新证据。

无论是什么原因导致的经济危机，对人们产生的冲击不应该从其数量级评估，而需要就其性质来进行判断。例如，一场金融危机可能给金融行业造成数以万亿美元的损失，同时因波及实体经济而造成大量赚取最低工资的劳动者丧失岗位。具体到个人，银行家和工人遭受损失的金额也不可同日而语，但是，在前一情形中，银行家损失的是资本所有者的钱，投资人面临的是资本收益的多少或有无，而在后一情形中，劳动者及其家庭失去的却是关乎生存的基本收入。

因此，在新冠肺炎疫情大流行时，低收入国家和低收入群体因不具备完善的医疗保障条件，更大的概率会首当其冲，生命和健康受到更大的威胁与伤害；进而，当疫情进入高峰期，"封城"和隔离等措施造成经济活动休止，脆弱的国家缺乏充足的资源和财力维系必要的检测、救治并保障居民基本生活，普通劳动者也更容易失去工作乃至收入来源，在暴露于生命健康风险中的同时陷入生活困境；而当经济开始复苏时，正如经济增长并不产生收入分配的涓流效应一样，普通劳动者的生活也不会随着经济的整体复苏自然而然回到正常轨道。

二　民生至上：中国经济复苏的第一位原则

（一）中国经济复苏的可能性轨迹

从底线思维出发，我们目前可以做出的判断是，中国经济几乎不再能够指望原来预期的 V 字形复苏轨迹。更具体来说，预期中国经济复苏，需要考虑到以下几种可能的模式，争取尽可能好的结果。

第一种可能性是，中国经济受到其他国家经济状况显著恶化以及世界经济严重衰退的影响，在经济恢复过程中步伐明显慢于原有预期。即便在相对好的复苏结果下，也会在原来预期的 V 字形轨迹基准上有所延迟，即需要有较长的时间在谷底或回升途中徘徊，形成一个 U 字形复苏轨迹。更不乐观的情形是可能形成一个"浴缸状"复苏，即受全球供应链断裂的干扰，在复工复产困难更大的假设下，经济景气处于谷底的时间将更久，进而经济增长回归潜在增长率的路程更长。

第二种可能性是，与全球新冠肺炎疫情的流行病学倒 W 形曲线相对应，中国经济的复苏在更大程度上受到世界经济衰退的拖累，形成较大跨度的 W 字形经济复苏轨迹，即复苏过程出现反复。甚至在更不乐观的情况下，特别是中国经济反复受到供给侧和需求侧的干扰，经济活动在回升过程中既需要花费更长的时间，甚至可能发生更多次的循环反复。

第三种可能性是，如果新型冠状病毒不像"非典"病毒那样在肆虐不长的一段时间之后便突然消失，而是病毒继续发生变异、在时间地点上呈现时隐时现的特征，以致新冠病毒肺炎成为一个长期存在、周期性出现的流行疾病，则可能形成一个与之对应的经济周期类型，经济增长也会遵循一个横向的 S 字形曲线波动。除非在各个国家都能形成群体免疫力，或者有效的疫苗研制成功，并且能够惠及世界上每个地方的每个人，否则世界和每个地区的经济活动从此会定时或不定时地发生停摆现象，中国经济相应也会受到影响。

（二）民生至上的中国式经济复苏

树立宏观经济政策的人文视角，坚持民生至上是经济复苏的中心性原则。中国抗疫工作并没有完成，将成为常态，因此，坚持我们的正确方针和卓有成效的工作机制十分重要。体现在复工复产、恢复经济活动的工作中，就是树立宏观经济政策的人文视角，坚持民生至上，因为每一个百分点失业率背后都是民生。一方面，中国有 6 亿人每个月的收入也就 1000 元，即大规模的低收入人群；另一方面，中国也拥有最多数量的中等收入人口。这是因为中国是一个人口大国，也是一个发展中国家，迄今仍然处于中等偏上收入国家行列的国情决定的。所以，无论是中等收入群体还是相对低收入群体，规模都是巨大的。

较大规模的低收入群体的存在，可以有两个政策含义。第一，这是一个具有很大市场潜力的群体，随着他们收入水平的提高，将加入中等收入群体行列，必然不断扩大消费内需，以更加可持续的需求动力拉动经济增长。第二，这部分人口也是拉低我国人均可支配收入的因素，其中一部分人可能还处在贫困状态，或者容易致贫或返贫，也可能是 2020 年打赢脱贫攻坚战的重点照顾对象。在新冠肺炎疫情的情况下会遭受较大的冲击，承受能力也较弱。因此，保障他们的就业和收入、基本生活，是最紧迫的政策取向。由于这个人群规模庞大，稳定他们的就业和民生，就能够做到"保居民就业"和"保基本民生"。

我们这次应对疫情以及疫情后复工复产的政策方向是非常正确的，总体上我们这次应对的政策，不适宜称为一揽子刺激政策，而是一个纾困救助政策组合。特别是中央提出的"六稳"和"六保"，都把就业居于首位。作为"之首"的含义，既是指其对民生的重要性，也是强调了这个问题的严峻性。

首先是遭受冲击的性质不一样。疫情一开始就带来供给、需求两端冲击，造成既不能生产也不能消费。在疫情得到控制，应该复工复产时，前期冲击出现滞后的负面效应。

其次是保就业与稳增长之间的关系不一样。传统思路是刺激经济以消除周期性失业现象。这一次首先要恢复居民的就业和收入。

最后是疫情是一种非市场外力冲击，导致劳动力市场失灵。因此，恢复就业需要政府以有形之手来推动。面对这场传播速度最快、感染范围最广、防控难度最大的重大突发公共卫生事件，各级政府要全力创造条件，救助小微企业、个体经营和各种形式就业，绝不能冷漠，各扫门前雪。要用最简单易行的办法，保障居民基本生活，吸纳农民工返城和失业群体再就业。

根据我国目前的流行病学曲线特征，从人口整体上是安全的。因此，全民核酸检测的目的要服务于复工复产，否则就把这个巨大的成本和机会浪费了。下一步，很可能全国很多地方都会选择全面核酸检测。各地在决策时要有明确的目标。做了检测的与尚未检测的要严格分开，以避免再次感染。已经检测证明安全的人群，要义无反顾地复工复产，不能再瞻前顾后。

三　中国抗击疫情和复苏经济的宝贵经验

（一）中国抗击疫情复苏经济的积极作为

新冠肺炎疫情不是产生于经济体系本身，完全是外部冲击。带来若干重要特点，理解这些特点有助于作出对于保就业和复苏经济更有针对性的决策。疫情一开始就带来供给、需求两端冲击，造成既不能生产也不能消费。在疫情得到控制，应该复工复产时，前期冲击出现滞后的负面效应。所以，经济复苏既不能指望外需也不能完全靠投资，居民消费需求需要以恢复就业为前提，按照先恢复就业，重新获得收入，进而有能力消费，为增长提供消费需求的次序，实现经济复苏。

密切关注流行病学曲线并不意味着只是等待。曲线不是注定的，也不应该以一成不变的方式去认识。各种防控措施本身就是改变曲线。立足于常态化就意味着不能等曲线完全见底后，再心无旁骛地复工复产。保持政策定力，对于疫情小幅反弹固然要充分重视，但不应该动摇复工复产的决心，不能停止复苏经济的步伐。要靠科学、精细化管理，不要简单化和一刀切。

中国坚持从以人民为中心的发展思想出发，以稳定就业、保障民生和实现脱贫目标为最高优先序，努力实现经济社会发展目标任务。中国长期向好的经济社会发展基本面没有变，也不会因为突发的疫情冲击而改变，即生产要素供给和生产率都不会受到长期影响。因此，总体完成预定的经济社会发展目标，特别是对于全面建成小康社会具有标志性的目标，仍然是必须付出巨大努力去争取的任务，不应有丝毫的懈怠。第一，一切旨在恢复经济活动从而刺激经济增长的宏观经济政策，都同时具有促进就业的效应，应最大化予以调动实施，并把就业优先政策纳入宏观政策层面。第二，针对失业成因中的结构性、摩擦性和周期性因素，有针对性地运用各种相关的政策手段降低整体失业率。第三，坚持社会政策托底，结余失业保险金除返还用于援企稳岗之外，还应该用于扩大支付范围，特别是覆盖未加入失业保险的返城失业农民工。此外，还需要通过设计更具普惠性、更直接快捷的项目，直接向受到疫情冲击的家庭支付现金。

可以预期的是，实现农村贫困人口全部脱贫的目标是可行的。党的十八大以来，全国农村贫困人口累计减少9348万人，也就是说在2012—2019年，每年实现脱贫人数都超过1000万人。2020年的任务是实现余下的551万农村贫困人口脱贫，按照近年来的脱贫速度，即便考虑到出现局部返贫现象可能加大工作难度，结合深入实施乡村振兴战略巩固脱贫成果，经过努力实现目标本来也是可以充分预期的。

在利用投资手段实施经济刺激的时候，需要充分汲取以往的教训，把握并守住几条不应突破的底线。要坚持发挥市场配置资源的决定性作用，避免产生不良债务积累和杠杆率的不合理提高，不产生新的低效产能和过剩产能，不发生系统性风险及其隐患的积累，不在污染防治攻坚战取得成效以及供给侧结构性改革成效方面发生任何倒退。

要防止经济增长形成对投资需求拉动的依赖，避免回归到传统发展方式上面。以往在宏观经济遭遇需求侧冲击时，投资对经济增长的贡献率就会显著提高，一旦形成对投资的依赖，需求结构就会失衡，从而损害经济增长的可持续性。长期以来，投资在中国经济增长的需求拉动中占据主导地位，经济快速增长也总是伴随着高投资率。并且，扩大投资常常被用来作为遭遇经济冲击（如出口下降）时的替代需求因素。

要把恢复经济活动、稳定增长速度、保障民生等紧迫任务与长期改革和发展的目标紧密结合。经济史表明，危机往往是充分暴露短板和结构性矛盾的时刻，相应地，应对危机和走出困境，也可以通过加快推进既定的长期改革和发展任务，在取得立竿见影效果的同时也可以产生长期可持续性的结果。新冠肺炎疫情暴露出的巨大经济社会短板和风险，最为突出的莫过于不完全或非典型化的城镇化。与此同时，城镇化预期也可以对中国经济社会长期发展做出重要的贡献。紧迫任务和长期目标的这一相会，就提出加快以农民工在城镇落户为核心的新型城镇化的紧迫任务。

要加快推进新型城镇化，加大农民工及家庭成员在务工所在城镇落户的户籍制度改革力度。这不仅可以从以上方面降低未来的经济社会风险，而且可以从增加劳动力供给、降低制造业成本、提高劳动生产率、提高基本公共服务均等化水平、改善收入分配和扩大居民消费等诸多方面，促进中国的经济社会长期可持续发展。目前我国常住人口城镇化率是60.6%，而户籍人口城镇化率仅为44.4%。也就是说，全国有2.27亿人口常住在城镇却没有取得城镇户口。这个人群的主体（高达76.7%）就是离开户籍所在乡镇外出务工的1.74亿农民工。这次疫情暴露出这种非典型化城市化的弊端，即在正常情况下返乡与返城造成的春运困难之外，额外地形成了人员密集流动产生的疾病流行风险、农民工不能及时返城复工造成的企业经营严重困难、农民工和农村居民收入大幅度减少，以及制造业供应链断裂乃至损坏的风险。

（二）中国抗击疫情、经济复苏的世界意义

除了新型冠状病毒本身演化显现出极端"狡猾"的特点及其造成疫情传播方式的特殊性之外，更重要的是，中国经济在世界经济中已经占有极大的比重，对世界经济的增长贡献独一无二，中国制造业在全球供应链中占据了中枢地位，中国经济增长正在进行动能的转换，以及世界处于更高全球化阶段的同时，逆全球化暗流也被推向高潮，等等。这些都对中国和世界应对这场经济冲击提出了前所未有的挑战。

这次疫情及经济影响事件的发生及其演变过程，也暴露出一系列在常态条件下被忽视的问题。例如，公共卫生应急响应体系、全球化条件下国家之间协同合作、紧急物资的储备和调运、制造业供应链的维护与修复等，都在疫情事件中遭到严峻的挑战。正因如此，经济学家需要进行更深刻的思考，以便提出对解决所面临各种困境的对策建议，同时能够未雨绸缪地预见将来。

在此次疫情暴发之前，经济全球化遭遇到单边主义、民粹主义、民族主义和贸易保护主义等各种政策倾向的冲击，美国也对包括中国在内的诸多重要经济体挑起贸易摩擦，并推动与中国经济及供应链脱钩。然而，疫情冲击下的世界经济挑战反而更加显示全球化的不可逆转性。中国经济在复苏过程中及之后，以自身的生产和供货维护并修复全球供应链，进而阻止经济全球化的倒退，将会发挥的作用是不可替代的。

在新冠肺炎疫情全球大流行趋势及其经济影响的不确定性中，坚定不移地推动中国经济率先复苏对世界经济复苏意义重大。作为世界第二大经济体以及经济增长最快的国家之一，近年来，中国对全球经济增长的贡献率高达 30% 以上。因此，在其他经济体乃至世界经济陷入衰退的情况下，中国经济的率先复苏不仅是中国自身的事情，对世界经济也绝不是零和博弈，而必然产生极为重要的正面溢出效应。更重要的是，中国经济迅速恢复到增长常态，对世界的意义也不仅仅是一个抽象的总量概念，而是可以从诸多重要方面对其他国家以及世界经济做出贡献。

Putting Life and Livelihood First

Cai Fang*

2020 is a particularly important year for China and the world. According to the blueprint of the 19th National Congress of the CPC, China will finish building a moderately prosperous society in all respects this year. The representative indicators of socioeconomic development, GDP and the income of urban and rural residents, will double between 2010 and 2020. Meanwhile, all rural residents falling below China's current poverty line will be lifted out of poverty. However, the coronavirus outbreak around the 2020 Spring Festival seriously disrupts normal social and economic activities, posing serious challenges to the attainment of the annual socio-economic development goals. The pandemic (the highest level of disease transmission defined by the WHO) has swept almost all countries and regions, wreaking havoc on the world's major economies. As a result, active isolation is imposed, leading to shrinking economic activities. Meanwhile, markets fluctuate due to active adjustment or panic, plunging the world economy into a steep recession.

In 2020, we have witnessed the ruling concept of putting life and livelihood first. Facing the pandemic, different countries adopt different approaches. Some Western countries resort to " the law of large numbers", trying to flatten the COVID-19 curves. It seems to be a scientific and feasible measure from a purely statistical point of view. However, because every case of infection is a case of health and life, state leaders who truly uphold the idea

---

* Cai Fang, Chief Expert of the National High-end Think Tank at the Chinese Academy of Social Sciences and Member of the Chinese Academy of Social Sciences.

of putting life and livelihood first will find it difficult to and will not accept the law of large numbers.

The idea is the guiding principle for China's fight against COVID-19 and its economic recovery. We don't take statistical risks such as "herd immunity". Rather, we persevere in taking necessary prevention and control actions at every stage, thus achieving an inverted V-shaped epidemic curve in a short time. We respect the law of the epidemic curve in our working steps, and at the same time, we have changed the curve with our own efforts.

I. Putting Life First: Fundamental Principle of China's FightAgainst Coronavirus

Although the coronavirus does "equal" harm to the life and health of all people, the basic health status between rich and poor countries and between different income groups are hugely different. So are the access to immunization, treatment, and rehabilitation, as well as the degree of the virus's economic impact and the endurance of different economies. Angus Deaton, the winner of the Nobel Prize in Economics, pointed out in his review of the history of pandemic and human response that the technology of preventing and treating an epidemic is usually transferred from the top of the social hierarchy to the bottom. Therefore, to this economist who revealed "deaths of despair" in America, not everyone is created equal in the face of the coronavirus.

Admittedly, in modern society, medical treatments are remarkably inclusive and accessible. But in the face of the coronavirus, whether billionaires and political elites in developed countries or unskilled workers living below the poverty line in developing countries, they have the same chances of infection and have to pay the price of health and even life after being infected. However, when it comes to whether there is a choice to avoid infection, what treatments are available after infection, whether the vaccine is accessible once it comes out, and especially the nature and degree of the impact of the pandemic, there are undoubtedly considerable differences be-

10

tween different countries and social groups. In the United States, many data show that African-Americans and Latino-Americans have a COVID-19 mortality rate several times higher than Caucasians. This is the latest evidence of the hypothesis that not all people are equal in the face of the pandemic.

No matter what causes an economic crisis, the impact on people should be evaluated not from its order of magnitude but from its nature. For example, the financial industry may lose trillions of dollars because of a financial crisis, but at the same time, a massive number of workers who earn the minimum wage will lose their jobs due to the impact of the crisis on the real economy. As far as individuals are concerned, the amount of losses suffered by bankers and workers cannot be mentioned in the same breath. While bankers lose the money of capital owners and investors lose the amount of capital gains, workers and their families are deprived of the basic income they live on.

Thus, during the coronavirus outbreak, low-income countries and groups are highly likely to bear the brunt, with a bigger threat to their health and life because they do not have good medical conditions. When the pandemic peaks and measures such as "city lockdown" and isolation bring economic activities to a halt, vulnerable countries run short of sufficient resources and finance to maintain necessary testing and fail to support and guarantee the livelihood of residents. Moreover, ordinary workers are more likely to lose their jobs and even sources of income, falling into a plight while being exposed to life and health risks. Just as economic growth does not produce the trickle-down effect of the income distribution, the life of ordinary workers will not naturally return to normal when the economy starts to recover.

II. Putting Livelihood First: Overriding Principle of China's Economic Recovery

(I) Possibilities of China's Economic Recovery

The bottom line thinking tells us that the Chinese economy can no longer have the originally anticipated V-shaped recovery. More specifically, the projection needs to consider the following possible models so as to strive for the best possible results.

The first possibility is that the Chinese economy will recover far slower than expected, as the economics of other countries are deteriorating significantly and the world economy in deep recession. Even economic recovery is good, there will be a delay in the expected V-shaped trajectory. In other words, it will stay around at the bottom or on the upswing side of the V shape for an extended period, forming a U shape. A worse scenario is a "bathtub-shaped" recovery. With the global supply chain being disrupted and the resumption work and production more difficult, the economic boom would be at the horizontal for a prolonged period, and thus it will take a much longer time for economic growth to return to the potential growth rate.

The second possibility is, corresponding to the inverted W-shaped curve of the COVID-19 pandemic, that China's economic recovery is encumbered by the global economic recession to a greater extent, forming a horizontally longer W shape, namely, repeated upturns and downturns. Even in a less optimistic situation, especially when the Chinese economy is frequently disturbed by the supply side and the demand side, the rebound will take longer, possibly with many fluctuations.

The third possibility is a horizontal S-shaped fluctuation if the coronavirus doesn't disappear suddenly after a short period of time like SARS and instead continues to mutate and appear and vanish from sight from time to time in different places so that the coronavirus persists for long as a periodic epidemic. Unless herd immunity can be achieved in every country, or an effective vaccine is successfully developed to benefit everyone in every corner of the world, global and regional economic activities will come to a standstill regularly or irregularly, which also affects the Chinese economy.

(II) Chinese-Style Economic Recovery that Puts Livelihood First

The central principle of economic recovery is to adhere to the macroeconomic policies with people and livelihood at the core. Since China has completed the anti-pandemic task, it is very important to adhere to correct policy and effective working mechanisms. When it comes to the resumption of work and production and the restoration of economic activities, it means to formulate macroeconomic policies with people and livelihood at the core because every percentage of unemployment will affect livelihood. On the one hand, China has a large lower income group, with 600 million people having a monthly income of barely 1, 000 yuan. On the other hand, China also has the world's largest middle-income group. This is because China is an upper-middle-income developing country with a huge population. Therefore, both middle-income groups and low-income groups are massive.

The existence of large-scale low-income groups has two policy meanings. First, they represent a population with great market potential. With a higher income level, they will enter the ranks of middle-income groups, and they will definitely expand domestic consumption and boost economic growth with more sustainable demand. Second, they are also the cause of China's lower per capita disposable incomes. Since some of them may still live in poverty or easily become impoverished or fall into poverty again, they could be the focus of this year's efforts to win the battle against poverty. Besides, they are vulnerable to the huge impact of the COVID-19 pandemic. Therefore, the most pressing issue is to guarantee the employment, income, and basic livelihood of this large population. If this target is met, we can achieve the goal of "ensuring the employment of residents and the basic livelihood".

We have a perfectly correct policy orientation toward the response to COVID-19 and the subsequent resumption of work and production. On the whole, these measures should not be called stimulus package but relief package. In particular, employment comes first in the central government's proposal to ensure "six priorities" and stability in six areas for steady economic momentum. Being defined as the "top priority" indicates its importance to livelihood and the seriousness of this issue.

Firstly, the nature of the impact differs. When COVID-19 broke out, both sides of supply and demand were affected, resulting in the suspension of production and consumption. When it was put under control and work and production were resumed, the early shock showed delayed negative effect.

Secondly, ensuring stability in employment is different from ensuring economic growth. The traditional approach is to stimulate the economy to eliminate cyclical unemployment. But this time, we must first restore the employment and income of residents.

Thirdly, the pandemic, as a non-market external force, leads to the failure of the labor market. Therefore, the recovery of employment entails the government's visible hand. In the face of this major public health emergency with the fastest spread, the widest range and the greatest difficulty in prevention and control, governments at all levels should make every effort to assist small and micro enterprises, the self-employed, and various forms of employment. Officials must not treat the matter with indifference. It is necessary to use the simplest ways to ensure the basic livelihood of residents, attract migrant workers to return to cities, and make the jobless re-employed.

According to the characteristics of the current epidemic curve in China, the population as a whole is safe. Therefore, the purpose of citywide nucleic acid testing should serve the resumption of work and production. Otherwise, this enormously costly opportunity would be wasted. It is likely that in the future, many places in China will choose comprehensive nucleic acid testing. Local authorities, however, must set clear goals in decision-making. Those who have been tested should be strictly separated from those who have not to avoid re-infection. People who have tested negative should return to work without hesitation.

III. China's Valuable Experience in Fighting COVID-19 and Reviving the Economy

(I) China's Vigorous Actions to Fight COVID-19 and Reinvigorate the Economy

The pandemic is not a problem inherent in the economic system but a purely external shock. Understanding its important characteristics enables us to make more targeted decisions to ensure stability in employment and revive the economy. When COVID-19 broke out, both sides of supply and demand were affected, resulting in the suspension of production and consumption. When it was put under control and work and production were resumed, the early shock showed delayed negative effect. As a result, economic recovery can neither count on external demand nor investment alone. Household consumption demand should be based on the premise of restoring employment and economic recovery should be achieved in the order of restoring employment, regaining income, restoring the power of consumption, and finally providing consumption demand for growth.

Paying close attention to the epidemic curve does not mean just sitting by and watching. The curve is changeable and thus should be understood in a flexible way. It is changed by various prevention and control measures. Adherence to normalization means that we should not wait for the curve to completely bottom out and then resume work and production. We also need to remain committed to the policy. In other words, while full attention should be paid to a slight epidemic rebound, the determination to resume work and production and restart the economy should never change. Besides, we should rely on scientific and refined management rather than simplistic and one-size-fits-all approaches.

China adheres to the concept of people-centered development and gives priority to stable employment, people's livelihood, and poverty alleviation to achieve the economic and social development goals. The fundamentals of China's long-term sound socio-economic development have not and will not be changed by the coronavirus outbreak. In other words, the pandemic will not have long-term implications for the supply of production factors and productivity. Thus we must, with the slightest indolence, manage to attain the scheduled socio-economic development targets, especially the historic goal of finishing building a moderately prosperous society in all respects. First, all macroeconomic policies aimed at restoring economic activities and stimulating economic growth help to boost employment and therefore should be vigorously encouraged and implemented to the maximum. At the same time, the policy of prioritizing employment should be included. Second, regarding the structural, frictional, and cyclical factors in unemployment, various related policies should be used to reduce the overall unemployment rate. Third, we should support economic policies with social ones. The surplus unemployment insurance benefits should be used to assist businesses and ensure steady employment. More importantly, it is important to expand the scope of the benefits to cover laid-off migrant workers who have not applied for the unemployment insurance. In addition, more inclusive, direct, and convenient projects should be designed to pay cash directly to families affected by the pandemic.

It can be expected that the goal of lifting all poor people living in rural areas out of poverty can be achieved. Since the Eighteenth National Congress of the CPC, 93. 48 million people living in rural areas have been lifted out of poverty, which means that every year from 2012 to 2019, more than 10 million people have escaped poverty. The task in 2020 is to lift the remaining 5. 51 million poor people in rural areas out of poverty. Considering the speed of poverty alleviation in recent years, even if the phenomenon that people in some rural areas will return to poverty makes the task more difficult, this target is still attainable by consolidating the achievements of poverty alleviation with the in-depth implementation of the strategy for rural revitalization.

In stimulating the economy with using investments, we need to fully grasp the lessons of the past and hold onto several bottom lines. It is important to give full play to the decisive role of the market in allocating resources and avoid the accumulation of non-performing debts and an unreasonable increase in the leverage ratio. We should refrain from producing new inefficient production capacity and overcapacity, accumulating systemic risks and potential hazards, and regressing to an early stage in pollution prevention and control as well as the supply-side structural reform.

It is necessary to prevent economic growth from becoming dependent on the demand generated by investment and avoid returning to the traditional development model. In the past, when the macroeconomy was impacted by the demand side, the contribution of capital formation to economic growth would increase significantly. But once the dependence on investment was formed, the demand structure would lose balance and thus damage the sustainability of economic growth. For a long time, China's economic growth has been chiefly driven by the demands deriving from investment, and rapid economic growth is always accompanied by a high investment rate. Moreover, expanding investment is often used as an alternative demand factor in the face of economic impact (such as falling exports).

The urgent tasks of restoring economic activities, stabilizing growth rate, and ensuring livelihood should be integrated closely with long-term reform and development goals. Economic history shows that a crisis is often a time when shortcomings and structural contradictions are fully exposed. Accordingly, resolving the crisis helps to complete long-term reform and development missions faster as well as producing long-term sustainable results. The most prominent socio-economic risk revealed by COVID-19 is incomplete or atypical urbanization. Urbanization is expected to make an important contribution to China's long-term socio-economic development. Because of the long-term goals, the urgent task of accelerating a new type of urbanization with urban residency for migrant workers at the core is put forward.

We need to speed up such urbanization and the reform of the hukou system so that migrant workers and their family members can register for permanent residence in urban areas. This can not only lower the future socio-economic risks but also promote long-term sustainable socio-economic development by increasing labor supply and productivity, reducing manufacturing costs, improving equal access to basic public services and income distribution, and expanding household consumption. The percentage of the population residing permanently in urban areas is 60. 6% , while the percentage of the population registered as permanent urban residents is only 44. 4% . In other words, 227 million people live in cities and towns without obtaining urban hukou, or household registration. A whopping 76. 7% of them (174 million) are migrant workers who have left their domicile for work in urban areas. The pandemic has exposed the drawbacks of this atypical urbanization: as traveling between urban areas and rural areas becomes very difficult during the Spring Festival under normal circumstances, there is a high risk of an epidemic caused by the intensive flow of passengers. As a result, it becomes extremely difficult to restart business operations because migrant workers cannot return to cities in time, leading to a substantial reduction in the income of these workers and rural residents as well as the possible rupture or even destruction of the manufacturing supply chain.

(Ⅱ) The Global Significance of China's Fight Against COVID-19 and Its Economic Recovery

Currently, the coronavirus is sweeping the world in an extremely "cunning" way, posing a threat to the world economy. On the other hand, the Chinese economy, which accounts for a huge proportion of the world economy, has a unique role to play in global economic growth, with the manufacturing industry occupying a central position in the global supply chain. In the face of COVID-19, the Chinese economy is witnessing the transformation of growth drivers, globalization is being taken to a higher level, and opposition against globalization is also reaching its peak. All these pose unprecedented challenges to China and the world as they need to tackle such economic impact.

With the pandemic and economic impact evolving, a series of problems neglected under normal circumstances have been exposed. For example, the coronavirus has seriously challenged the public health emergency response system, the cooperation between countries in the era of globalization, the storage and transportation of emergency supplies, and the maintenance and repair of manufacturing supply chains. Therefore, economists need to think harder to put forward measures against various difficulties and plan ahead.

Before the coronavirus outbreak, economic globalization was hit by various trends, such as unilateralism, populism, nationalism, and trade protectionism. The US also has trade friction against many major economies, including China, and tried to decouple the American economy and supply chain from China. However, the challenges facing the world economy merely demonstrate that globalization is irreversible. During and after recovery, the Chinese economy will play an irreplaceable role in maintaining and repairing the global supply chain with its production and supply, thus preventing the retrogression of economic globalization.

As we are not certain about the global pandemic trend and its economic impact, unswervingly helping the Chinese economy to recover first is of great significance to the world economic recovery. As the world's second-largest economy and one of the fastest-growing economies, China has contributed more than 30% to global economic growth in recent years. Therefore, when other economies and the world economy have plunged into recession, helping the Chinese economy to recover first is neither China's own business nor a zero-sum game for the world, because it is bound to produce extremely important positive spillover effects. More importantly, such effects will not only expand the size of the world economy but also contribute to the world economy and other economies in many important aspects.

人类命运共同体

COVID-19 新冠病毒肺炎：一次对人类命运共同体的考验

颇钦·蓬拉军（Bhokin Bhalakula）

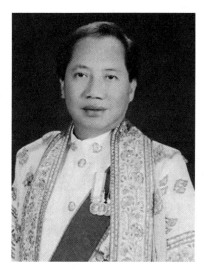

自 2012 年以来，我一直在关注并研究中国提出的关于构建人类命运共同体的提议。在 2019 年访华期间，我在中国许多地方作的大部分演讲都是针对该提议的。自邓小平时代起，中国共产党根据中国的现实国情和对未来的愿景，创造性地解释并贯彻了马克思主义理论，提出了"中国特色社会主义"和"社会主义市场经济"等概念。这一举措不仅是为了为中国人民带来和平、幸福和安定，而且推动了整个国际社会朝着和平、绿色、可持续发展等目标迈进。同时，中国提议在协商、合作、双赢和相互尊重的前提下共同努力消除贫困。四川文理学院马克思主义学院的林世珍（音译）总结道，人类命运共同体是对马克思主义的继承和发展，是从互联和发展的角度来审视世界，是利用互联的积极方面来推动一国的发展。然而，这一概念又十分复杂，我们需要做进一步的研究才能更好地理解。

中国领导人和中国共产党构建人类命运共同体的倡议是对中国自身和世界的一份承诺。这一概念体现了中国的意愿和决心：中国不仅

颇钦·蓬拉军，泰中文化经济协会会长，泰国前副总理。

要与他国和平共处，还要与他国通力合作，共同应对和解决复杂的世界经济和其他问题，因为当今世界没有一个国家能够独善其身。

目前以单边主义为核心并由美国主宰的世界秩序正面临新理念的挑战。新的世界秩序以多边主义为前提并以中国提出的"一带一路"倡议为手段，以人类命运共同体的建立为标志。

针对中美贸易摩擦，哥伦比亚大学杰弗里·萨克斯（Jeffey Sachs）说过，"这场贸易摩擦并不是在中美两国间展开的，而是一场美国与国内大型企业的战争。这些公司大多在日进斗金的同时，却未能向自己的员工支付足够体面的工资。美国的巨富和商业领袖在推动减税、争取更多垄断权力，并将资产向海外转移，以赚取更大的利润。与此同时，他们却拒绝支持任何使美国社会更加公平的政策"。

可以说，实现人类命运共同体并非一日之功，现在世界各地还存在着冲突、战争、恐怖主义、饥荒、经济和社会不公等诸多问题。此外，我们还面临全球变暖、自然灾害以及此次的新冠肺炎疫情等问题。新冠肺炎疫情是全人类的敌人，其威力足以摧毁人类和地球，但似乎我们总是会忽视这一点。

新冠肺炎疫情刚开始出现时，许多国家似乎认为这只是中国国内的事情。为此，一些国家尝试安排撤侨专机，一些国家领导人，尤其是西方国家领导人当时也错误地估计了局势，低估疫情的严重性，甚至少部分国家指责中国故意隐瞒病毒发源地、病毒威胁和感染人数等信息。

事实表明，中国始终秉持开放、透明、负责任的原则，及时公开相关信息，分享应对疫情和治疗经验。需要特别指出的是，中国还尽其所能，为其他受疫情影响的国家提供医疗和其他物资。这一举动得到了 2020 年 4 月 2 日发布的《世界政党关于加强抗击新冠肺炎疫情国际合作的共同呼吁》的称赞。

截至目前，世界上大多数国家和人民都将新冠病毒肺炎视作人类共同的敌人，应动员全部力量与之抗争。大多数国家正在开展合作，共同控制疫情暴发、分享经验并开展联合研究，以研发出应对病毒的有效药物和疫苗。从中我们看到全球公共卫生命运共同体的建设，而这次合作也将为在未来构建人类命运共同体打下基础。

当然，人类命运共同体发展之路并非一帆风顺，沿路布满荆棘坎坷，有些国家仍对基于霸权的陈旧思维和态度抱残守缺，为一己之私利，而将公共卫生问题政治化。

指责任何组织或国家都无益于缓解疫情扩散的现状。相反，我们应该明白，没有任何一个人或国家愿意看到疫情发生在自己的领土上，也不想将其用作武器摧毁他国。现在，新型冠状病毒已在全球范围内扩散开来，疫情也不可能在短期内结束，能有效抑制病毒的药物或疫苗也不可能很快出现。如果不与他国和国际组织开展合作协调，仅凭一国之力难以独善其身，更无法战胜病毒。

现实是，我们必须联合起来，将这次病毒危机转化为机遇。首先要在全球范围内建立应对此次疫情的医疗标准。其次，各国应紧密协作，确保世界各国经济、社会发展获得令人满意的结果。

联合国、世界卫生组织、国际贸易组织、世界银行、国际货币基金组织和所有国际实体必须与所有国家紧密合作，摒弃偏见，无视某些政客的政治把戏，最终赢得与新型冠状病毒的战争，进而建立以人类命运共同体为核心的全球新秩序。（董方源翻译）

原文：

COVID-19：The Test of The Shared Future for Humanity

Bhokin Bhalakula[*]

I have followed and studied the Chinese concept about the importance of building of a community of a shared future for mankind since 2012, and

---

* Bhokin Bhalakula, Former Deputy Prime Minister, Thailand.

during my visits to many places in China last year, 2019, most of my speeches were dedicated to the said proposal. The Communist Party of China (CPC) has, since Deng Xiaoping, used the phrase "Socialism with Chinese characteristics" and "socialist market economy", by interpreting and implementing Marxism theory in line with the current situation and future trends to bring peace, happiness and stability not only to the Chinese people but also to push the international community towards peace, green and sustainable development and the eradication of poverty on the basis of negotiation, collaboration, win-win solution and mutual respect. Shizen Lin of College of Marxism, Sichuan University of Arts and Science, Dazhen, concluded that a community of a shared future for mankind is the inheritance and development of Marxism to see the world from the perspective of interconnectedness and development, and to use the positive aspects of interconnectedness to promote the development of one's country. However, this concept is a complex one which deserves further research for a better understanding.

In my view, the proposal of the Chinese leaders and the CPC to build a community with a shared future for mankind is both an internal and external commitment for China and the world. The concept has reflected the Chinese will and intention not only to live peacefully with other nations but to stick and work together to face and solve complicated world economic and other problems and difficulties, because no country can stay protected by only taking good care of itself.

In a word, the present world order focused on unilateralism and dominated by USA is being challenged by the new world order through the building of a community with a shared future for mankind initiated by China, with the Belt and Road Initiative and multilateralism as its means.

I do agree with Professor Jeffey Sachs of Columbia University, with regard to the trade friction between USA and China, in stating that "the real battle is not with China but with America's own giant companies, many of which are taking in fortunes while failing to pay their own workers decent wages. America's business leaders and the mega-rich push for tax cut, more monopoly power and offshoring anything to make a bigger profit while rejecting any policies to make America's society fairer. "

I realize that it is not really easy to achieve such a goal since everywhere in the world today there have been conflicts and wars, terrorism, famine, starvation, economic, social inequalities and etc. Besides, we are also facing global warming, natural disasters and particularly pandemic diseases. The latter are the real enemies of mankind and can destroy our earth and our human race, but it seems that we were always unaware of it.

With the coming of COVID-19, in the beginning it looked like many countries thought that it was a problem for China. Some nations tried to get its citizens back from Wu han as quickly as possible. Many world leaders, especially in the western bloc, played down the situation and underestimated the epidemic. Some accused China of concealing the facts regarding the origin of the virus and its dangers, as well as the number of infected people.

Finally, China has shown that it has adopted an open, transparent and responsible attitude to disclosing the related information in a timely fashion, by sharing its experiences on response and patient treatment, and in particular providing medical and other supplies, to the best of their ability, to other affected countries, as praised by "A Joint open letter from world political parties concerning Closer International Cooperation against COVID-19" announced on April 2, 2020.

At present, I think that most nations and people regard COVID-19 as an enemy of humanity and we must forge our force and ability to fight against and to defeat it, and I have confidence that most nations will cooperate in containing the outbreak, share experiences and conduct joint research to develop specific medicines and vaccines to cope with the virus. This time I believe that we will see a global community with a shared future for public health, which will be a stepping stone to the building of a community of a shared future for mankind.

Nevertheless, this road map is not covered with a soft carpet, but in fact is covered with thorns since leaders of some countries still have an obsolete vision and attitude based on hegemonies, and have politicized the public health issues for their benefit.

To blame any organization or any country does not help alleviate the pandemic situation. In fact, we can simply understand that no one or no country wanted to see this kind of epidemic occur on its territory or to use it as a weapon to destroy others. At present, the virus has spread all over the world and it is unlikely that the outbreak will be over soon or that we will have developed a vaccine or medicine to effectively contain the outbreak in immediate future. It is evident that a single country cannot be safe from or fight against the virus without collaboration and coordination with the rest of the world and all International Organizations concerned.

Therefore, we have to be united, turn this virus crisis into opportunity, first, to establish the health care standard against this pandemic globally, and second, to collaborate and cooperate closely to ensure that world and national economic and social development can go on with satisfactory results, even though it is seriously affected by COVID-19.

The United Nations, the World Health Organization, the World Trade Organization, the World Bank, the International Monetary Fund and all International Entities involved must work closely with all countries, without bias and disregard any kind of politics played by some politicians to win the final victory against COVID-19 and to further set up a new world order focused on building a community of a shared future for mankind.

将全世界命运共同体作为资本全球化的一种方案

何塞·路易斯·森特利亚·戈麦斯
（Jose Luis Centella Gomez）*

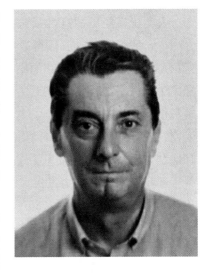

我们应当牢记，所谓的具有资本主义性质的新自由主义全球化的衰落在 COVID-19（新冠病毒肺炎）引发危机之前就已经存在了，因为我们能越来越清晰地看到仅仅依靠以单极世界为基础的国际关系体系无法解决人类的诸多问题，在这一体系中，大国攫取利益是以损害落后国家的利益为代价的，也就是所谓的零和理论。

事实上，本次疫情正在加剧这种衰落，并引发了新的危险，因为新自由主义全球化已经对人类造成了不利影响，而一些资本主义思想家关闭边境、阻碍国际贸易和加剧单边主义国际关系等防卫方案可能会使情况更加糟糕。

面对这种思想，我们应当提议，新自由主义全球化的危机可以让路给一种以国家关系的多边化和横向化为基础的新型全球治理方式，从而发展一种互惠的公平贸易，摒弃零和理论，让所有国家互利共赢，还要在国际秩序和国家制度中做出巨大改变。

---

* 何塞·路易斯·森特利亚·戈麦斯，西班牙共产党主席。

　　中华人民共和国国家主席习近平提出的构建人类命运共同体的设想就完全符合这种新型全球治理方式的理念，它将实现共同目标的合作意愿和努力结合起来，让世界上所有的居民都能有权享有体面的生活，并集中力量一起对抗一些紧急情况，比如人类正在经历的危机。

　　构建人类命运共同体不仅有助于我们通过相互合作和资源共享来为当前的紧急情况找到最快的出路，还能发展出有利于全人类的全面可持续的共享安全理念，从而帮助我们避免目前这种情况再次发生。

　　没有人能否认当今世界上所有的国家和地区之间都存在完全的相互依存关系，问题是能够从互惠合作的层面来面对这种相互关系，通过合作来共享资源和技术进步，以共享的方式来增加利润，还要制定明确的规则来帮助和保护弱小贫困国家免受大国和发达国家的侵害。

　　人类正在经历的这种紧急危机向我们表明，危机没有国界，也不分洲界，我们必须加强国际合作，发挥联合国的作用，推行《联合国宪章》中包含的价值观和原则，因为如果没有一个像联合国这样的完全民主和权威的机构，就无法进行全球治理，因为它能控制其他国际经济机构，让它们对遭受紧急情况影响较大的国家发挥更大的作用。因此，国际经济合作必须经历重大变革才能建立起新的规则，才能更好地利用经济来改善那些受危机影响的人们的生活质量。

　　近几年来的生产力发展、技术进步和医学上的重大发现让我们现在有能力面对像目前的危机一样的紧急情况，要构建人类命运共同体，只需要结束既没有控制措施又没有道德约束的新型自由主义市场，同时制定规则和控制措施来加强为摆脱危机和普遍利益而提出的经济政策之间的关系，始终参考国家的领导路线来捍卫共同利益。

　　通过国际机构来巩固世界各国之间的新型政治、经济和文化关系框架所要解决的基本问题是设计一个能解决当前危机所造成的后果的"重建地球"的伟大项目，一个拥有充足的经济支持和一些能避免不公正、新殖民主义或环境恶化等情况的明确规则的"伟大项目"。

　　为了使人类有一个共同的"伟大项目"，中华人民共和国政府与许多国家和来自全球的经济组织合作制定的倡议强有力地呈现在我们眼前，我指的是"一带一路"倡议，因为目前，这对于克服全球将遭受的经济危机可能会大有帮助，对最脆弱和最不受保护的国家将会产生更深的影响。

"一带一路"倡议已经成为历史上最大的国际合作项目，我们提议全球所有国家都将该"倡议"视为共享机遇，这样才能协调各个项目和资源，将其用于世界经济的复苏，因为全世界的生产力正在遭受的停滞毫无疑问会对其产生影响。

综上所述，我们不得不提出在当前阶段应加强各种倡议、论坛和会议，使国际社会向不同政府施加压力，要求它们搁置分歧并关注具有普遍意义的项目，这将带领我们进入那个伟大的"人类命运共同体"，它对于我们面对这种全球紧急情况的后果是必不可少的。

因此，最重要的是我们民间社会、公民协会、经济组织应意识到必须从我们的经历中汲取经验，应该明白只有在全球所有居民之间建立一种合作和协作的关系，我们才能从当前我们正在遭受的紧急情况中走出来，要更加融洽，更加团结，更加坚定，跨越国界，跨越种族，所有人联合起来，以全人类的共同命运为目标构建一个"伟大共同体"，我们定能够成功面对未来可能给我们带来的挑战。（徐璞玉翻译）

原文：

The Community of Common Destiny as An Alternative to Capitalist Globalization

Jose Luis Centella Gomez *

It is important to bear in mind that the decline of the so-called Neolib-

---

* Jose Luis Centella Gomez, President, Communist Party of Spain.

eral Globalization, capitalist in character, precedes the crisis caused by the COVID-19. It has been more and more evident that the problems of humanity cannot be solved with a system of international relations based on a unipolar world, in which the profits of the great powers are achieved at the expense of the losses of the less developed states, in what is called the theory of the zero sum.

What has happened is that the crisis which is provoking the Pandemic is aggravating this decadence. This is bringing about a new danger, because if the Neoliberal Globalization was already negative for humanity, the alternative that some capitalist thinkers are defending of closing frontiers, hindering international trade, and aggravating the unilateral character of international relations, can be even worse.

With all of this in mind, a proposal can be raised that allows this crisis of Neoliberal Globalization to give way to a new World Governance based on multilateralism and horizontality in the relations between States, which develops a fair trade of mutual benefit in which everyone wins. that they bury the zero-sum theory and make great changes in the international order.

The proposal made by the President of the People's Republic of China, Xi Jinping, to build a Community of Common Destiny that joins forces and wills in order to achieve cooperation. This cooperation can lead to common goals so that all the inhabitants of the World can have the right to a dignified life and join forces to fight together against emergency situations such as the one humanity is currently experiencing.

Building a Community of Common Destiny is what can allow not only to facilitate a faster exit from the current emergency situation through mutual cooperation and the possibility of sharing resources, but it can also help us to prevent situations like the current one from repeating themselves, developing a concept of integral and sustainable shared security for the benefit of all humanity.

No one can deny that in today's world there is total interdependence between all countries and territories; the question is to be able to face this interrelationship from mutual cooperation that manages to share resources and technical advances in order to multiply the gain in a shared way, by elaborating clear rules that help and protect the weakest and most vulnerable States from the aggressions of the most powerful and developed States.

To begin with, an emergency crisis such as the one humanity is experiencing at the moment shows us that crises do not respect borders or continents, making it necessary to strengthen international cooperation by promoting the role of the UN. In order to recover the use of the values and principles contained in its Founding Charter, because there cannot be a Global Governance without an institution that represents it with a fully democratic and representative character and that has control over the international economic institutions, to make them more useful to the countries that are going to suffer the most from the emergency situation. In this sense, the international economic cooperation must undergo great changes to establish rules that allow a better use of the economy to improve the quality of life of those who are affected by the consequences of the crisis.

In these times, the development of the productive forces, the technological advances, and the medical discoveries allow us to face emergency situations like the present one. It is only necessary to finish with a neoliberal market that has neither control nor morals to constitute a Community of Common Destiny, and develop rules and controls to promote the relation between the economic policies that are raised to leave the crisis mindful of the general interest, always under the direction of the State as reference of the defense of the common good.

The basic question to consolidate a new political, economic and cultural frame of relations between the States of the world, from some international institutions, is the design of a great project of Reconstruction of the Planet that faces the consequences that the current crisis is causing. A Great Project that counts on sufficient economic support and clear rules to avoid situations of injustice, neocolonialism, or environmental degradation.

In this goal of providing humanity with a common Great Project, the initiative that has been developed for some time by the Government of the People's Republic of China in collaboration with several States and economic organizations from all over the world appears with great force. I refer to the Belt and Road Initiative because at this time it can be of great use in helping us overcome the economic crisis that the whole world is going to suffer and which will affect the weakest and most unprotected countries most profoundly.

The Belt and Road Initiative is already the largest international cooperation project in history. The proposal is that this Initiative be seen by all the countries of the world as an opportunity to pool projects and resources to be dedicated to the reactivation of the world economy that no one doubts will be affected by the paralysis that production is suffering throughout the world.

Considering all these arguments, we must propose that at this time it is necessary to intensify all the initiatives, forums and meetings so that the international community can put pressure on the different governments to set aside differences and pay attention to projects of general interest, which would lead us to that great Community of Common Destiny of Humanity, which is necessary to face the consequences of this world's emergency situation.

Thus, it is important that the Civil Society, the Citizens Associations, and the economic organizations become aware of the need to learn from the experience we are living and understand that only establishing relationships, cooperation and common work among all the peoples of the World, can allow us to get out of this emergency situation, which we are suffering, more united, more in solidarity, more convinced, beyond borders, beyond races, all together we can successfully face the challenges that the future may bring, shaping a Great Community with a Common Destiny for all Humanity.

"人类命运共同体"理念：
应对疫情最适合

萨达特·曼苏尔·纳德利
(Sayed Sadat Mansoor Naderi)*

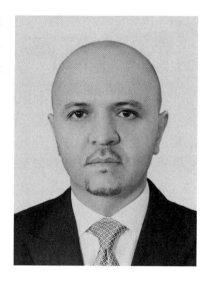

"新冠病毒肺炎"于2020年年初传播到世界各地，引发了自1918年"西班牙流感"之后的又一场全球疫情。

各国纷纷关闭企业，居民被禁足在家。各国政府承诺投入数万亿美元以维持经济。各国央行已大幅降息，并推出了大规模的量化宽松计划，各国政府也正在启动大规模的宽松财政政策。许多西方国家及远东各国都注意到，中国、日本与韩国有经济实力对其卫生部门及经济利益大量投入。

不幸的是，非洲、亚洲其他地区及拉丁美洲的发展中国家却是这场疫情中最脆弱的地区，因为它们的国家卫生基础设施状况不佳，财政能力不足，无法在新型冠状病毒蔓延期间启动其经济引擎。

暂缓病毒传播的一些关键指标是勤洗手与保持一定的社交距离。但在一些贫穷国家，用水本身就是问题，更别提洗手了。许多社区的人们生活在贫民窟条件下，区域内本就拥挤不堪，这也给保

---

* 萨达特·曼苏尔·纳德利，阿富汗伊斯兰共和国城市发展与住房部前部长。

持个人社交距离构成了不可能完成的挑战。对这些较贫穷的国家而言，客观上减轻压力的是病毒对老年人或本身就有基础病的人群更易致死，而欠发达国家同富裕国家相比，其人口构成中年轻人口所占比例更高，老龄人口所占比例更低。此外，欠发达经济体的贫困人口多居住在农村及城市地区，而据了解，病毒在人口密集的城市中传播更盛。

"新冠病毒肺炎"暴发带来的影响将是政府债务以惊人的速度增加，政府支出加大，还会导致货币宽松政策的增加，而税收则会减少。为了平衡预算，各国政府或许会加税，特别是对富人加税，或是对大公司征税。而这很有可能会再一次导致过去就曾出现过的经济大萧条。

病毒还将带来的影响是促使各国将目光转向国内，并自行生产绝大部分生活必需品。这将会导致消费品价格的上涨，并将导致国际贸易的缩减，从而造成全球范围内创新与财富创造的减少。

当今世界在经济上是相互联系的，仅仅一件简单的产品也会具有依赖性，在各大洲及多国拥有多条价值链。举例来说，汽车生产的供应链涉及并依赖多个大洲及国家以生产出最终产品。

新型冠状病毒对不那么富裕的社会产生的有害影响要比对富裕社会的影响大得多。在当前这场疫情及封锁期间，蓝领岗位受到的冲击最大。简单列举一下，工厂车间工人、酒店业与零售业的工人受到的冲击最为严重。而白领职工仍然可以在家隔离远程办公，比如记者与高管。

过去几十年间，贸易与移民为整个世界都带来了经济福祉。这种情况主要发生在诸如中国、印度这样人口稠密的国家。不幸的是，因为疫情大流行，移民与贸易也将受到影响。由于各国不愿再签发签证，这又会反过来影响贸易、商业及投资活动。

如果我们有一种共同的、"全人类共命运"的方法，这一新型冠状病毒就不会失控。各国就可以从一开始就共同努力，互相帮助，彼此扶持，以阻止病毒扩散开来，同时考虑在各国境内采取预防措施应对病毒。

一些举措，比如信息共享、勤洗手、自我隔离、封锁，以及包括呼吸机、口罩、检测试剂盒与防护服在内的特殊医疗设备，对于抗击病毒的传播都是十分关键的。

在阻止新型冠状病毒在国内的传播方面，中国一直是一个好榜样。中国立即采取严格措施封锁了武汉，重点防止病毒向全国其他地区传播。其结果是更少的人员伤亡与更小的经济影响。当中国开始抗击病毒时，世界上其他国家还曾质疑过其方法，今天，中国却成为所有正在遭受苦难的国家的榜样。

中国的"人类命运共同体"理念在支援并提供人力资源以及向世界其他国家运送医疗物资方面也被证明是积极有效的，中国向意大利派遣医生以提供支持，并向他国运送了呼吸机、口罩及防护装备。在此情形下中国所采取的积极行动都在拯救生命中发挥了关键作用。

人类命运共同体的理念非常适合类似新型冠状病毒这样的危机情景。对付这个看不见的敌人，最好的办法是全世界共进退，对彼此友好并相互扶持，从错误中吸取教训，成功实施好的实践做法，以抗击新型冠状病毒的传播。

除此之外，各国与各大实验室之间应实现信息共享，以便研发疫苗。为尽早达成这一点，各国应在区域及全球范围内共同努力，与各自研发中心一道寻找到疫苗，以对抗谁都不希望发生的世界各地进一步的反复感染浪潮。各国、各地区想要恢复到过去的水平，即使不需要几十年也需要好几年的时间。在贸易、商业、经济及货币政策上通过二十国集团、联合国等大集团共同进退，将对经济发展恢复繁荣产生最有效的影响。

各国应在区域范围及全球范围内设立不同的基金以实现经济稳定，从而为不那么富裕的社会成员创造就业机会。

新型冠状病毒对劳动力市场的负面冲击已经产生了最大影响。全球已有数亿人失业，美国目前的失业人数已达 2200 万人。这是美国历史上失业率上升幅度最大的一次，自 2007—2008 年的国际金融危机以来，美国创造的所有就业岗位均已被抹除。欧洲、日本、中国还有印度也都面临同样的境遇。

新冠病毒肺炎是一场流行病，它也是看不见的敌人，对经济的供需双边都造成了最大冲击。全世界应共同解决这一问题。"人类命运共同体"的理念最适合应对这一场疫情。它要求全球各大平台都能具备集体思维。

疫情之后的世界将不再是我们所熟知的世界。对航空与酒店等众多行业的负面影响或许很难消除，人们对于旅行必要性的看法将更为凸显。视频会议与居家办公将成为常态，而前往商业中心出差开会则将成为过去。

上网课，当前的这一新概念或许将被广泛接受，政府与家长可能会更倾向于这种教育方式。父母会更多地参与到孩子的学习当中，感到更有控制力。

各行各业将受到鼓励选择人工智能，机器将取代人力资本成为主导资源。

疫情后的社会影响主要体现在全球范围内人们见面打招呼、聚会以及社交的方式都将与过去有所不同。

每个国家都受到了冲击，尤其是各自的医疗卫生部门，未来对医疗基础设施、疫苗研发的投资与准备工作都将有所增加。未来各国还会努力自行生产绝大部分重要的医疗设备与装备。诸如卫生部门等领域的贸易壁垒或将增加，以保护国内产业。这或许将对创新与价格竞争力产生负面影响。

为避免后疫情时代的负面影响，世界各国领导人应搁置分歧，以合作的方式应对当前疫情。我们已经经历了新型冠状病毒的传播，影响了我们当中的每一个人。如果全世界采取团结一致的应对举措抗击疫情，在未来对于气候问题及其他相关流行病的应对上，这将成为我们这一代人最普遍的经验学习曲线。大家异口同声地回应并行动。

这个看不见的敌人无视壁垒，不分肤色、种族、性别与宗教，也不分地域、贫富和老幼——它是我们人类一个看不见的敌人。对我们共同的社会与人类这一种族而言，一个有着明确愿景的集体路径才是前进的唯一办法。（杨莉翻译）

原文：

A Community with a Shared Future for Mankind: the Most Appropriate Concept to Respond to the COVID-19

Sayed Sadat Mansoor Naderi *

The dangerous virus COVID-19 has spread throughout the world creating a global pandemic since the Spanish flu of 1918.

States have shut down businesses and populations are in lock down. Governments have promised trillions of dollars to keep the economy on life support. Central banks have cut their interest rates dramatically and have launched massive quantitative easing schemes. Governments are easing fiscal policy on a massive scale. Many western countries along with Far East Asia, noting China, Japan and South Korea have the financial muscle to spend enormously for the benefit of their health sectors and economies.

Unfortunately other developing countries in Africa, Asia and Latin America are the most vulnerable due to their poor state of health infrastructure and financial incapacities, unable to kick start their economic engines during the coronavirus contagion.

Some of the key indicators to stave off the spread of the virus are washing hands regularly and social distancing. In poorer countries, access to water is an issue, let alone washing hands. Many communities live in slum con-

---
* Sayed Sadat Mansoor Naderi, Former Minister, Housing and Urban Development, Afghanistan.

ditions and within crowded areas, which creates the impossible challenge to social distance oneself. However, the good news for the poorer nations is that the virus tends to be deadly for the elderly and those with existing medical conditions. Less developed nations tend to have a higher population of young people, and less elderly in comparison to their richer counterparts. Also poorer populations in less developed economies tend to reside in rural and urban areas. It is known the virus thrives in highly populated cities.

The affect of COVID-19 outbreak will find government debts increasing at a phenomenal rate, spending and monetary easing will also increase, tax revenue will decrease. In order to balance the budget, governments may either increase taxation especially on the rich or place levies on big corporations. This is likely to result in another great depression seen in the past.

The effect of the virus will make countries to look inward and self produce most of their essential goods. This will result in price increases of consumer items and will see a reduction in international trade resulting in less innovation and less wealth creation globally.

The world currently is so commercially interconnected that a simple product has many value chains and dependencies across different continents and countries. The example of a car production's supply chain involves and relies on many continents and countries to create the finished product.

The detrimental impact of Coronavirus upon societies less well off, is much bigger than that of the rich and wealthy. During the current pandemic and its lockdown, the blue collar jobs have been impacted the most. Factory floors, the hospitality industry and retail workers to name a few have been the worst hit. White-collar workers are still functioning from home in isolation remotely such as journalists, executives.

The past several decades, trade and immigration has resulted in economic well being for the world as whole. This has largely been seen in highly populated countries like China and India. Unfortunately due to the pandemic, immigration and trade will be affected. As countries become reluctant to issue visas, in turn impacts trade, commerce and investment.

If we had a collective approach and shared "a future for mankind" approach, this coronavirus would not have got out of control. Countries could have worked collectively in helping and supporting one another to prevent the spread of the virus from the outset, whilst at the same time consider precautionary measures within their own borders to tackle the virus.

Some of the measures like sharing information, washing your hands, self isolation, lockdown, specific medical equipment like ventilators, masks, testing kits and protective clothing are key factors to fight the spread of the virus.

China has been a good role model in stopping the spread of coronavirus within its borders. China took immediate strict measures by locking down Wuhan province and focused on preventing the spread of the virus to the rest of the country. This has resulted in lower human casualties with less economic impact. When China started combatting the virus, the rest of the world had doubts about their approach, today China has become a role model for all countries currently suffering.

China's approach for shared mankind has also proven to be effective in supporting and providing human capital by sending doctors to Italy for support, as well as shipping medical equipment like ventilators, masks, and protective gear to the rest of the world. Such positive action in these circumstances has played a crucial role in saving lives.

The concept of community with shared value for mankind fits perfectly with a crisis scenario like coronavirus. The best approach in fighting such an invisible enemy is for the world to have a collective approach, be kind and supportive to each other and learn from mistakes and apply good practices for successful implementation to combat the spread of the coronavirus.

Alongside this, information between countries and laboratories should be shared so a vaccine can be found. To do this earlier than later, countries should work collectively regionally and globally with their research and development centres, to find a vaccine to combat further unwanted repeated waves of infection around the world. Countries should work together within their economic policies and commerce to get the world economy prosperous and growing again. It will take years, if not decades for countries and regions to get back to where they were. A collective approach on trade, commerce, economic and monetary policies through various blocks like G20 and UN, would have the most effective impact towards economic development back to prosperity.

Countries regionally and globally should create various funds to create economic stability to create jobs for the less wealthier members of society.

Already coronavirus's negative shock on the labour market has had the biggest impact. Hundreds of millions of people have been made unemployed across the globe, with the US currently standing at 22 million lost jobs. This is the biggest rise of unemployment in its history, every job that was created in the US since the 2007 and 2008 financial crisis has been wiped out. Europe, Japan, China and India are all facing the same fate.

Coronavirus is a pandemic, it's an invisible enemy which has had the biggest shock on both the demand and supply side economically. The world must therefore tackle it collectively. The concept of community with shared value for mankind fits tackling this pandemic the best. It requires collective thinking on various global platforms.

Post Pandemic, the world will not remain as we know it. The negative impact affecting many sectors such as aviation and hospitality may not recover, and people's perceptions on traveling for necessity will become more pronounced. Virtual meetings and home working will become the norm whilst traveling to a hub to meet for business will be a thing of the past.

Virtual learning, the new concept of today may become widely accepted and preferred by the governments and parents across the educational spectrum. Parents will feel more in control and will become more involved in their child's learning.

Industries will be encouraged to opt for artificial intelligence where machinery will be the dominant resource as opposed to human capital.

Social impact of the post pandemic with the way people greet, gather and socialize will be different across the globe.

Every country has received their shock particularly in their health sector, future preparation and investment in health infrastructure and research and development towards vaccines will be increased. Countries will also try to self produce most of their vital medical equipments and kits in the future. Trade barriers in sectors like health may increase to protect their domestic industries. This may negatively effect innovation and price competitiveness.

In order to avoid the negative impact of the post pandemic, the world leaders should put aside their differences and approach this pandemic cooperatively. We have already experienced the spread of the virus on the world in a space of 3 months affecting every person in our communities. If the world approaches this pandemic with a collective united response, it will be the most prevalent experimental learning curve of our generation, for our future climate and other health related pandemics. Acting and responding, with one voice together.

This invisible enemy knows no barriers, colours, race, gender, religion, geography, rich, poor, young or old—its an unseen enemy against our human race. Requiring a collective approach with clear vision for our shared community and mankind is the only way forward.

后疫情时代的人类命运共同体建设

赛义德·哈桑·贾维德（Syed Hasan Javed）[*]

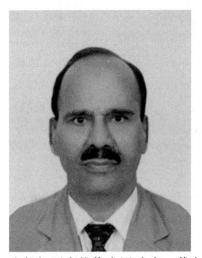

2019 年 12 月，中国成为全球最早遭受新冠病毒攻击的国家之一。中国随即向世卫组织、包括美国在内的相关国家和地区通报相关信息。在确定该病毒为新冠病毒后，中国与世卫组织共享了病毒基因序列，并决定对疫情最严重的武汉进行封城。经过三个月英勇的努力，中国战胜了新冠病毒，于 2020 年 4 月 8 日解除了对武汉的封锁。中国身处抗击新冠病毒的第一线，为世界各国树立了榜样。没有任何国家能像中国政府、像与中国人民紧密团结的中国共产党这样，在如此短的时间之内动员民众、调配物资。中国应对危机的速度和纪律彰显了中国在社会管理、治理体制和民众动员方面的固有优势。中国对疫情信息的披露一直是开放、透明、负责的。联合国、世卫组织，以及多国首脑与疾控专家都对中国迅速、有力和高效的反应给予了高度评价，称其为全球抗疫作出了贡献。美欧国家虽然坐拥无与伦比的医疗资源和技术，却创下全球最多的确诊病例和死亡人数记录。中国已呼吁各国提高全球公共卫生意识。疫情结束后，世卫组织应本着开放、透明和包容的态度，适时评估各国应对新型冠状病毒的

---

　* 赛义德·哈桑·贾维德，巴基斯坦国立科技大学（伊斯兰堡）中国学研究中心主任。

反应，总结其中的经验教训并提出针对性建议，避免悲剧重演。

中国向美欧提供帮助，为全球合作树立了榜样

在抗击新型冠状病毒的紧要时刻，中国基于自己"人类命运共同体"理念的朴素文化传承，向一些发达国家和发展中国家提供了紧急帮助。中国的积极思维是：在所有国家安全之前，任何国家都不能在公共卫生危机面前独善其身；国际社会比以往任何时候都更加需要团结和合作；人类的共同敌人是病毒。中国与美国不一定非要彼此为敌，而应该携起手来，共同抗击疫情；国际社会应当摒弃意识形态和政治制度的差异，携手保卫人类文明。秉承这一精神，中国政府、非政府组织、企业及个人向美国提供了倾情帮助。据中国官方消息，截至 2020 年 5 月 6 日，中国各省、市、机构和公司已向美国 30 个州、55 个市捐赠了 960 万只口罩、50 万箱拭子、30.59 万副医用和其他手套、13.35 万副护目镜以及其他医疗物资。中国海关统计数字显示，自 3 月 1 日至 5 月 5 日，中国已向美国提供了逾 66 亿只口罩、3.44 亿副外科手套、4409 万套防护服、675 万副护目镜，以及近 7500 台呼吸机。中国还向意大利、西班牙、希腊、匈牙利、塞尔维亚等欧洲国家提供了宝贵支持，这些国家在其他欧洲国家对其关闭边界后，被迫独自面对新冠肺炎疫情。中国政府还向亚洲、非洲和拉丁美洲的一些国家供应了大量的口罩、扫描仪、呼吸机及其他医疗物资和设备，帮助其抵御疫情。

与中国的做法相反，美国右翼政客和政府却将新冠肺炎疫情视为在意识形态和地缘政治上攻击中国的借口。美国还指控俄罗斯与中国"沆瀣一气"。美国似乎决意要在一个变革的世界中重新挑起不得人心的冷战"遏制论"，以遏制中国的和平崛起。事实是，在新冠肺炎疫情暴发之前和期间，西方媒体网络始终充斥着反华宣传。例如，武汉封城与中国政府的举措被西方社交和网络媒体描述为"对自由和人权的侵犯"。很明显，无论中国说什么或做什么，美国及其少数盟友都把中国视作是一个"威胁"。西方媒体上日复一日的涉华负面报道，反映了西方学界对中国崛起的深层忧虑。西方思维似乎依赖于招"鬼"，即制造想象的威胁。这与近年来国际知名民调机构所做的民意调查是背道而驰的。这些调查已经显示，中国民众对政府的支持率

和满意率高居世界首位，中国民众对政府的抗疫表现打分最高。在中国外交部 2020 年 5 月 9 日发布的长达 30 页的文件中，中国政府有力地驳斥了美国主要政客和政府官员关于新型冠状病毒的 24 个谎言、影射和宣传。

后疫情时代，"一带一路"合作重要性将愈发凸显

中国提出的"一带一路"倡议，旨在通过重启"丝绸之路经济带"和"21 世纪海上丝绸之路"，将亚欧大陆与非洲、美洲整合起来，打造"人类命运共同体"。"一带一路"倡议计划通过六大走廊建设，实现中国与亚洲、欧洲和非洲国家互联互通，预计完成的基建、联通和能源项目总值将达 1.2 万亿美元。价值 620 亿美元的（尚在建设当中的）中巴经济走廊是中国这一划时代倡议的"旗舰"项目。在亚洲、非洲、拉丁美洲和部分欧洲，中国被视作是追求和平崛起的稳定力量。值此艰难时刻，中国通过共享自己的抗疫知识、技能、物资和器械，为国际合作树立了杰出的榜样。亚欧人民梦想在"一带一路"基础设施中增加一条"丝路卫生走廊"，如同绿色走廊、数字走廊、教育走廊和文化走廊一样。

中国始终坚信，不同文明和制度之间可以和平共处，可以相互借鉴，可以共同进步。新型冠状病毒为各国社会、经济、贸易、政治和国际关系打造了一个全新的环境。病毒将继续带来重大伤亡（这取决于人类能在多短时间内找到可靠的疫苗并上市）。因此，"一带一路"国家应在医疗卫生、数字/网络贸易、电子商务、精准扶贫、债务免除、加强团结等方面进一步加强合作。这一点十分重要。在这一进程中，中国完全可以发挥示范和引领作用。中国扮演全球领导角色的时刻到了，世界对此期待已久。

结 论

无论美国极右翼政党、学者和官员如何污蔑，世界上绝大多数爱好和平的人都不会相信他们关于新型冠状病毒的谎言。中国的"一带一路"倡议代表着全球化的下一阶段。无论西方媒体如何宣传，历史

的进程也不可逆转。"一带一路"将是未来世界的"获胜联盟"。中国有能力领导这个世界。千百年来（而不是几十年来），由于西方的掠夺性思维：地缘政治主导、贪婪、剥削和暴力，我们的世界曾饱受战争冲突、环境毁灭、社会倒退和支离破碎的蹂躏。然而，要重塑理性和对话、恢复全球团结，就需要所有渴望拯救人类大家庭的国家的共同努力。最好的情况是，如同历史上的大多数时候一样，这个通向更美好世界的具有划时代意义的转折将通过进化而非战争来实现。也许这一代人足够聪明，能够沿着和平、发展的道路打造人类命运共同体。"一带一路"已经成为打造21世纪命运共同体的最流行的外交词汇。对广大发展中国家和新兴国家而言，中国通过改革而实现的和平崛起发展模式极具吸引力。（王文娥翻译）

原文：

Building a Community of Shared Destiny for Mankind：In Post COVID-19 Era

Syed Hasan Javed[*]

Introduction

China was among the first countries hit by COVID-19 in December, 2019. It started immediately sending timely updates to World Health Organization (WHO), relevant countries including the US and regions. After iden-

---

* Syed Hasan Javed, Director, Chinese Studies Centre of National University of Sciences and Technology.

tifying the virus as COVID-19, it shared the genetic sequencing information of the virus with the WHO and imposed lockdown on Wuhan, the worst hit by the Virus. After three months of heroic efforts to overcome the challenge the lockdown was lifted on April 8, 2020. China set an example as the first line of defense against the coronavirus. No country can replicate the exemplary pace of mobilization in men and material for the control of coronavirus as the Chinese government, Communist Party in solidarity with the Chinese masses were able to do. The pace and discipline with which China handled this crisis brings to light several in built strengths of the Chinese society, governance system and the masses China has been open, transparent and responsible in releasing information on the epidemic. Heads of the UN, WHO and many countries as well as medical experts in disease control all spoke highly of China's swift, strong and effective response which contributed to the global fight. Despite having unrivalled medical resources and technology, the US and European nations have continued registering the highest numbers of confirmed cases and fatal cases in the world. China has called for enhanced global public health preparedness. The WHO should assess global response to COVID-19 in an open, transparent and inclusive manner at an appropriate time after the pandemic is over. It can summarize experiences and shortfalls in the global response and propose, avoiding repetition.

China Sets Example of Global Cooperation: Send Assistance to US and Europe

Even when China was fighting relentlessly the coronavirus, it rushed assistance to several Developed and Developing nations in line with its pristine cultural heritage, that believes that "all human societies share the same destiny". It has a positive mindset that no country can guarantee its absolute security in public health alone, until all countries are safe. The international community therefore needs solidarity and cooperation more than ever. The common enemy of the humanity is the virus. China and the US need not become enemies of each other rather should join hands to fight the epidemics. The international community need to put aside all the differences in ideology and political system, to protect human civilization. In this spirit, the Chinese government, Non-Governmental Organizations (NGOs), Enterprises and individuals extended whole hearted assistance to even the United States According to official Chinese sources, as of May 6, 2020, Chinese provinces, cities, institutions and companies have donated more than 9. 6 million masks, 500000 boxes of testing reagents, 305900 pairs of medical and other gloves, 133500 pairs of goggles and other medical supplies to 30 states and 55 cities in the US. According to Chinese customs statistics, from March 1 to May 5, China has provided more than 6. 6 billion masks, 344 million pairs of surgical gloves, 44. 09 million sets of protective gowns, 6. 75 million pairs of goggles and nearly 7500 ventilators to the US. China also extended valuable support to several countries in Europe such as Italy, Spain, Greece, Hungary, Serbia etc. who were left alone to face the COVID-19 Pandemic, with closing of borders by their European compatriots. The Chinese government extended generous assistance to several Nations in Asia, Africa, Latin America through supply of masks, scanners, and ventilators as well as other medical material and equipment to cope with the COVID-19 pandemic.

In contrast, the right wing politicians and official US government have used the COVID-19 Pandemic in ideological and geo-political terms for attacking China. The US even accused Russia for collaboration with China. The Americans appear determined to revive the discredited "Cold War" template of "Containment Theory" in a somewhat transformed world, aimed this time at thwarting China's peaceful rise. It is a fact that even before, during and current COVID-19 crisis, one thing that remained constant, has been anti China propaganda in the Western media networks. For example, the Wuhan lockdown and Chinese government measures were described as "attack on Freedoms and Human rights" in Western social and electronic media. It is evident that irrespective of what China says or does, the United States and its few so-called allies treats China as a "Threat". The Western media is full of negative stories on China, day in and day out, reflecting the deep frustrations within the Western intelligentsia over China's rise as a global power. It appears that the Western mindset survives on creating "Ghosts" as imaginary threats. This is despite the surveys by well-known international poll agencies in the past few years which have shown that the Chinese people's support to and satisfaction with their government, ranks the top in the world. China ranked the highest in terms of epidemic response rated by its people. The Chinese government has refuted effectively all the 24 lies, insinuations and propaganda made by leading US Politicians, Officials with respect to COVID-19, in a 30 Page document issued on 9 May, 2020 by the Ministry of Foreign Affairs.

Belt and Road Initiative Cooperation Gains Added Significance in Post COVID-19 Era

China's Belt and Road Initiative (BRI) aims to build a "Community of Shared Destiny" for mankind by integrating the Euro-Asiatic Regions with Africa and Americas, through reviving the "Silk Route Economic Belt and the 21st Century Maritime Silk Route". The BRI envisions construction of Six Corridors connecting China with 65 countries in Asia, Europe and Africa. The total worth of the Infrastructure, Connectivity and Energy Projects planned to be completed is worth US $ 1. 2 trillion. China Pakistan Economic Corridor (CPEC) worth US $62 billion (and still evolving) is the "Flagship" Project of this epoch making Chinese Initiative paradigm. Across Asia, Africa, Latin America and parts of Europe, China is seen as the Stabilizer, seeking a peaceful rise. China has set a remarkable example of international cooperation even in times of great difficulties, sharing its knowledge, expertise, material and machines to cope with the COVID-19 Virus which is now a global Pandemic. The BRI countries have benefited immensely from China's timely and liberal medical assistance. The people in the Euro-Asiatic world dream to establish a "Silk Route Health Corridor" just like Green Corridor, Digital Corridor, Education Corridor or Cultural Corridor to complement Infrastructure loaded BRI.

China always believes that different civilizations and systems in the world can coexist in harmony, learn from each other and achieve progress together. The COVID-19 has created a qualitatively new environment for every society, economy, trade, politics and international relations. Depending on how soon a credible vaccine can be found and commercialized, the virus will continue to take a heavy toll. It is hence important for all BRI states to promote closer cooperation in healthcare sector, digital /online trade, E-Commerce, targeted programs for poverty reduction, debt waivers and strengthening global solidarity. China may lead by example. History teaches us that the moments of crisis are also time for new great powers. It is China's hour to provide global leadership the world has been waiting for long.

Conclusions

Irrespective of what the US extreme right wing parties, intellectuals, officials say, the peace loving majority population of the world is not ready to believe in its false COVID-19 narratives. The Chinese Belt and Road Initiative is the next phase of globalization. Irrespective of what the media in the Western societies may say, the march of history cannot be reversed. The BRI is the future "Winning Coalition" of the world. China has ability to lead the world, devastated by wars and conflicts, Environment destruction, Social decay and breakdown in human solidarity for not decades but centuries because of the predatory Western thought process of geo political domination, greed, exploitation and violence. The restoration of sanity, dialogue and revival of universal solidarity will however require collective efforts by all Nations eager to salvage the human family. It is better that such an epoch making transition to a better world, is achieved by evolutionary process instead of through wars, as had been most of the time in history. May be, the present generation will be smart enough to build a Community of Shared Destiny by following the path of peace and development. The BRI has become the most popular cliché of diplomatic Parleys, for building a Community of Shared Destiny in the 21st century. The Chinese development model of peaceful rise by undertaking reforms appeals, to the vast majority of people in the developing and emerging world.

疫情彰显更高眼界更阔视野的
人类命运共同体

许庆琦（Koh King Kee）*

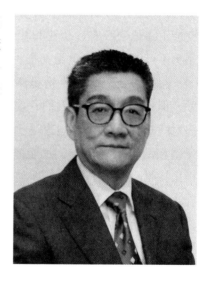

如果此前许多人对人类命运共同体的认知只是一个模糊的概念，新冠肺炎疫情无疑给人们上了生动的一课：病毒是人类的共同敌人，病毒袭击人类，不分肤色、种族、宗教或国家；在疫情面前，全世界人民休戚与共，风雨同舟。

历史上每一次的瘟疫大流行，都改变了人类历史的发展轨迹，新冠病毒肺炎大流行也势必如此。2020 年 4月 3 日美国前国务卿基辛格在《华尔街日报》撰文指出，"新冠病毒肺炎大流行对人类健康的攻击可能是暂时的，但它所引发的政治和经济动荡可能会持续几代人，新冠病毒肺炎大流行将永远改变世界秩序，疫情之后，世界将会变得不一样"。著名历史学家《人类简史》作者尤瓦尔·赫拉利在《金融时报》发表的长文《冠状病毒之后的世界》中强调，"我们这一代人正面临人类最大的危机，各国政府应对这危机的决定，不仅影响我们的医疗系统，也将影响我们的经济、政治和文化"。他说，疫情过后"风暴将过去，人类将继续存在，我们大多

---

* 许庆琦，马来西亚新亚洲战略研究中心理事长。

数人仍然将活着，但将生活在一个不同的世界"。

近年来欧盟国家民粹主义兴起，美国特朗普总统上任后实行美国优先政策，接连退出巴黎气候协定、联合国教科文组织、万国邮政联盟等国际条约与组织，设立关税壁垒，掀起了一股逆全球化浪潮。大流行期间，各国为阻止病毒蔓延，保护国民安全，纷纷关闭边境，禁止医药和医护用品出口。因此，多国学者担忧新冠病毒肺炎大流行将加速世界逆全球化的发展。哈佛大学肯尼迪政府学院教授斯蒂芬·沃尔特认为，新冠肺炎疫情"将加强民族主义，创造出一个不再那么开放、繁荣与自由的世界"。英国皇家国际事务研究所所长罗宾·尼布莱特指出，"新冠肺炎疫情可能是压垮经济全球化的最后一根稻草。疫情正在迫使政府、企业和社会加强长期应对经济孤立的能力，世界几乎不可能回到21世纪初那种互利共赢的全球化状态"。

然而，新冠肺炎疫情虽激起了不少专家学者对经济全球化的反思，但也同时提醒了人们，瘟疫无国界。在这高度互联互通的世界，面对病毒，没有一个国家是孤岛，可以独善其身。全世界人民必须守望相助，团结合作，才能战胜病毒。基辛格在其评论文章中坦诚指出，"没有一个国家，即使是美国，能够通过单纯的国家努力战胜这种病毒"。几百年来，全球治理都是由西方国家主导，以西方价值观作为衡量世界是非好坏的标准。疫情导致世人对全球化的反思，但无意间也给中国倡议的人类命运共同体全球治理理念带来新契机。

新冠病毒肺炎大流行不会终结全球化，只是终结了由西方主导的全球化。新冠肺炎疫情将改变世界秩序，疫情过后，世界将进入构建人类命运共同体的新全球化时代，一个体现人文关怀的新全球化时代。作为世界工厂，中国深入参与全球产业链。疫情期间中国的经济活动停摆，冲击了全球供应链。疫情之后各国政府和跨国企业基于国家安全战略与运营风险考量，必将对各自的生产和供应体系有所调整。但中国多年建立起来的国内完备的产业体系所带来的效益与效率，以及其庞大的国内市场，是其他国家难以复制的。因此，疫情之后中国仍将会在全球供应链扮演举足轻重的角色。疫情促进了科技的应用和创新发展，改变了人们的生活习惯、学习和工作方式。人工智能和互联网颠覆了传统世界，人与人之间的关系不再取决于空间距离。我在新华社的专访中说："世人将会因新冠大流行重新思考全球化，但人与人之间的联系是无法切断的，新冠肺炎疫情提醒世界走向人类命运共同体，人与人之间的内心感情、文化交流等互联关系将更加紧密，而不仅仅是贸易与投资。"中国传媒大学人类命运共同体研究院院长李怀亮教授在《从全球化到共同体时代》一文的结论这么写道："人类命运共同体理念是中国处理国际事务的指导思想。在这次抗击疫情的过程中，中国正在实践着这一理念，疫情改变着世界，疫情之后，人类命运共同体意识将具有更为广泛的国际共识，成为国际社会主流话语体系。"

新冠肺炎疫情暴发后，中国政府迅速采取了果断、强势、有效的干预措施以阻止病毒从"震中"蔓延扩散，史无前例的对一千万人口的武汉封城，切断对外交通，城内强制集中隔离病患，及时阻止一场可能因春节期间大量人员流动而造成的瘟疫大灾难。中国发挥制度优势，及时动员全国人民，调派4万余名医护和志愿人员奔赴一线服务，以"中国速度"建立了两家新冠病毒肺炎应急医院和十多家方舱医院。中国人民付出了巨大代价，在不到三个月内以血泪和汗水阻击病毒蔓延，成功阶段性地控制了疫情。中国在抗击疫情中显示出来的体制优势，世人有目共睹。许多遭受新型冠状病毒肆虐的国家，也纷纷仿效中国阻击疫情蔓延的强势措施。中国抗疫取得的成果以及对其他受到新型冠状病毒重创国家的支援，彰显了一个负责任大国的担当，受到了国际组织如联合国、世卫、国际货币基金等以及各国领导人的高度评价和赞赏。

但也有别有用心的西方媒体和个别政客，借病毒污名化中国，扭曲疫情，借此抹黑中国形象，诋毁中国。但这一切都掩盖不了事实，改写不了历史。在人类与疾病抗争的历史长河中，中国对此次新冠病毒肺炎大流行做出的牺牲与贡献，必将留下重要的篇章。正如《中美能否避免修昔底德陷阱》一书作者格雷厄姆·艾里森所说的："如果中国政府展示出了确保其公民的最基本人权——生命权——的能力，而一个民主的、分权的政府却还纠缠不清，那么反对中国过去采取的措施的异议，在许多人看来都是酸葡萄。"西方自由主义体制的缺陷在疫情中显露无遗，相对中国的担当，美国没有挑起领导世界各国抗击新型冠状病毒的责任。特朗普对疫情大意轻敌，病毒袭击美国后，却推诿责任，嫁祸中国。因此，新冠大流行必将削弱美国作为世界霸主的地位，但即便如此，疫情不会是美国的"苏伊士时刻"，西方将继续主导全球治理体系。

疫情给了中国难得的历史机遇。人类命运共同体作为新全球化时代的国际共识，中国要以更高的眼界和更阔的视野彰显其时代性，超脱"讲中国的故事"的框框，以"胸怀世界，心系天下"的大国风范表述人类命运共同体；从全球的角度，构建一个既受到世人普遍接受，又具有中华文化色彩的配套世界观与价值观。中华文化源远流长，博大精深，5000年的历史沉淀不乏足以世界共享的智慧结晶。"天下"是中华文化传统的世界观。"大道之行也，天下为公"是儒家思想中的理想世界，习近平主席在多次演讲中提到《论语》中的这句话。这里的"天下"指的是全世界，"公"则是指人类命运共同体。"天下"不强调国界，宣扬大同世界的理念，正是共同体所追求的目标，是具有中华文化色彩的国际主义。"仁得天下，不仁则失。""仁"是中华文化伦理思想中最核心的价值理念，是中国人的基本价值观。"仁"是人类的共同价值，最能体现人类命运共同体的人文关怀。基督教的"博爱"是西方价值观的基础，伊斯兰教教义强调"公正、平等"。而"仁"则两者皆有，是中华文化最具代表性的价值理念。"仁"与"天下"这两个古老的中华文化传统理念，必将随着人类命运共同体成为国际社会主流话语体系而发扬光大。

中国的近代史，历经苦难，饱受天灾人祸和内战外辱之害。然而每一场苦难都使得中华民族更加坚强，战胜病毒克服疫情之后，中华民族必将在伟大复兴的道路上跨一大步，为人类命运共同体做出更大的贡献！

译文：

Community with a Shared Future for Mankind: Higher and Broader Vision Amid COVID-19 Pandemic

Koh King Kee *

Previously a vague concept for many people, the Community with a Shared Future for Mankind is undoubtedly a clear and vivid idea in the wake of the coronavirus outbreak: viruses are the common enemy of humanity as they attack humans, regardless of their color, race, religion or country; in the face of the pandemic, people all over the world stand together, sharing weal and woe.

Every former pandemic has changed the course of history. So will the COVID-19 outbreak. Former Secretary of State Henry Kissinger wrote for The Wall Street Journal on April 3, 2020 that "While the assault on human health will be temporary, the political and economic upheaval it has unleashed could last for generations. The coronavirus pandemic will forever alter the world order. The reality is the world will never be the same after the coronavirus." In his article, The World After Coronavirus appearing in the Financial Times, famous historian Yuval Noah Harari, author of *Sapiens: A Brief History of Humankind*, emphasized that "Humankind is now facing a global crisis. Perhaps the biggest crisis of our generation. The decisions people and governments take will shape not just our healthcare systems but also

---

* Koh King Kee, President of the Center for New Inclusive Asia.

our economy, politics, and culture. " "The storm will pass, humankind will survive, most of us will still be alive — but we will inhabit a different world," he added.

Recent years we have witnessed the rise of populism in EU countries and the surge of deglobalization. Since taking office, US President Donald Trump has implemented the America First policy, erected tariff barriers, and withdrawn successively from the Paris Agreement, UNESCO, the Universal Postal Union, and other international treaties and organizations. To stop the spread of the virus and protect national security during the pandemic, countries around the world have closed their borders and prohibited the export of medicines and medical supplies. This is why many scholars worry that COVID-19 may accelerate deglobalization. Stephen M. Walt, a professor at the John F. Kennedy School of Government at Harvard University, believes that COVID-19 "will reinforce nationalism and create a world that is less open, less prosperous, and less free. " Chatham House Director Robin Niblett pointed out that " COVID-19 could be the straw that breaks the camel's back of economic globalization. Now, COVID-19 is forcing governments, companies, and societies to strengthen their capacity to cope with extended periods of economic self-isolation. It seems highly unlikely in this context that the world will return to the idea of mutually beneficial globalization that defined the early 21st century. "

While the coronavirus has prompted many experts and scholars to reflect on economic globalization, it also reminds people that a pandemic disease respects no borders. In this highly interconnected world, no country can totally stay safe from the virus. Only when people all over the world work together to help each other can we defeat the coronavirus. As Henry Kissinger frankly pointed out, "not even the US can in a purely national effort overcome the virus. " For centuries, global governance has been dominated by Western countries, with Western values as a yardstick by which to measure the world. As the world ponders over globalization, COVID-19 is inadvertently bringing new opportunities for China to advocate the global governance concept of a Community with a Shared Future for Mankind.

The pandemic will not terminate globalization; rather, it ends the West-dominated globalization. The world order will be changed and after the coronavirus, the world will usher in a new globalization era, a Community with a Shared Future for Mankind, that embodies humanistic care. The world factory, China, will play a greater role in the global industrial chain. Economic activities came to a standstill in China during the coronavirus outbreak, exerting an impact on the global supply chain. After the pandemic, governments and multinationals will adjust their production and supply systems based on national security strategies and operational risks. However, it is difficult for other countries to replicate China's huge domestic market and the benefits and efficiency created by China's comprehensive domestic industrial system over the years. Hence China will still play a pivotal role in the global supply chain after the pandemic. Because of COVID-19, the application and innovative development of technology have been enhanced, changing people's living habits, study, and work styles. AI and the Internet have transformed the old world, removing the spatial distance that limits the interpersonal relationship. Recently, I said in an exclusive interview with Xinhua News Agency: "While the world will rethink globalization due to the pandemic, the connection between people won't be severed because COVID-19 reminds the world to move towards a Community with a Shared Future for Mankind. People will become closer and there will be stronger cultural exchanges, in addition to trade and investment exchanges." In his article From Globalization to the Age of a Community with a Shared Future, Professor Li Huailiang, Dean of the Institute for a Community with Shared Future at the Communication University of China, concludes, "The concept of a Community with a Shared Future for Mankind is the guiding principle for China to handle international affairs. It was practiced by China in its fight against the coronavirus outbreak. The pandemic is reshaping the world. After COVID-19, the concept will have wider international recognition and become the mainstream discourse of the international community."

Following the coronavirus outbreak, Chinese authorities swiftly took decisive, stringent, and effective measures to contain the spread of the virus from the "epicenter" of Wuhan, a city with a population of 10 million people. The entire city was placed on lockdown, external traffic was cut off, and centralized isolation of patients was imposed. All these moves, which had never been attempted before, timely prevented an epidemic disaster that might be caused by a massive flow of people during the Spring Festival. Using its institutional advantages, China mobilized its people in time, dispatching more than 40, 000 medical staff and volunteers to the front line and establishing two COVID-19 emergency hospitals and over ten purpose-built field hospitals at the "China speed". The Chinese people paid a big price, but in less than three months, they successfully curbed the spread of the virus and put it under control. China's institutional advantages in that combat are obvious to the world. The strict yet effective measures of China were also followed by many other countries ravaged by the virus. China's achievements in the combat and support to other countries plagued by coronavirus demonstrate its role as a responsible major country and are highly commended by leaders of many countries and international organizations such as the United Nations, the WHO, and the IMF.

Nonetheless, some Western media and individual politicians with ulterior motives vilified China and distorted the pandemic to tarnish China's image and defame China. But all these cannot cover up the truth or rewrite history. In the long history of fighting against diseases, what China has sacrificed for and contributed to the fight against the pandemic will surely become an important chapter. As Graham Allison who wrote *Destined for War: Can America and China Escape Thucydides's Trap?* pointed out, "If an Chinese government demonstrates competence in ensuring its citizens' most basic human right—the right to life—as a democratic, decentralized government flounders, objections to the measures China has used to do so will sound to many like sour grapes." The defects in Western liberalism are fully revealed by the coronavirus. Compared with China's strong sense of duty, the US fails to assume the responsibility of a leader in the global fight against COVID-19. As coronavirus swept across America because Donald Trump played down its effect, the president, however, shirked his responsibility and shifted the blame onto China. Therefore, the pandemic will definitely weaken the position of the US as a world hegemony. Yet it will not be America's "Suez Moment", and the West will continue to dominate the global governance system.

But it will give China a rare historic opportunity. As the Community with a Shared Future for Mankind represents an international consensus in the era of new globalization, China should show its epochal nature with a higher and broader vision, go beyond the frame of "telling Chinese stories", and express the major-country style of "caring about the world". It should create a world outlook and values universally accepted by the world and with Chinese cultural elements. The long-standing, profound Chinese culture, with a 5000-year history, has abundant wisdom to share with the world. "World community" is the traditional world view in Chinese culture. "When the great way prevails, the world community is equally shared by all." Such an ideal world of Confucianism stated in The Analects of Confucius is mentioned by President Xi in many of his speeches. Here, "the world community" refers to the whole world and "equally shared by all public" denotes the Community with a Shared Future for Mankind. With no emphasis on national boundaries, this is the goal pursued by the Community and internationalism with Chinese cultural characteristics. "It is with benevolence that the world becomes one community". "Benevolence" is the core of Chinese cultural ethics and part of the fundamental values of Chinese people. It is the universal value of mankind, which best reflects the humanistic care of the Community with a Shared Future for Mankind. Christian "fraternity" is the foundation of western values, while Islamic doctrine emphasizes "justice and equality". The concept of "benevolence" is a combination of both. It is also the most representative value of Chinese culture. "Benevolence" and "World Community", two ancient concepts of Chinese culture, are bound to spread across the world as the Community with a Shared Future for Mankind becomes the mainstream in the international community.

In modern times, China suffered from not only natural and man-made calamities but also civil war and foreign invasion. But every tribulation only makes the Chinese nation stronger. After defeating COVID-19, the nation is bound to take a huge step forward on the road to great rejuvenation and make a greater contribution to the Community with a Shared Future for Mankind!

抗疫合作昭示"人类命运共同体"
建设的必由之路

吴白乙*

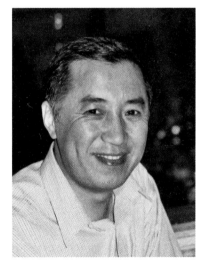

"历史每过一段就划下一个分水岭。"2020 年的全球新冠病毒肺炎大流行，冲破了我们共同生活星球上的自然和人为制度界限，对全人类的健康和安全形成了前所未有的严峻挑战。这是一场历史性的大考。随着各国抗击疫情斗争的深化，其答案必将越来越接近时代发展的本真，也是我们翻过这道分水岭，迈向疫后共同发展的共识与动能。

首先，在经济高度全球化的背景下，人类流动迁徙的自由程度远超过 20 世纪，密布于全球的资金链、产业链、供应链、信息链以至于人际关系链已自然浑成。它们一方面是造成疫情广为传播的客观前提，另一方面也造成大疫之前"地不分南北，人不论贫富，国无谓强弱"，各方都是受害者、抗争者以及未来胜利者的共同身份。正如谭德塞总干事在第 73 届世界卫生大会上讲话指出的那样，"疫情提醒我们，尽管彼此有诸多差异，但我们同属一个人类社会，团结在一起才会更强大"。

其次，抗疫斗争在全球展开以来，各国守望相助，相互支援，分享数据信息、诊疗经验以及卫生救急物资，科学界、企业界和社会组

* 吴白乙，中国社会科学院欧洲研究所原所长、研究员。

织也围绕疫苗和相关药物开发等开展交流，体现了人类在重大灾难面前的良知和理性。目前，抗疫斗争仍未有穷期。由于各地的疫情峰值期有先后之分，任何先走出危机的国家无法独自全面恢复经济和社会生活，受疫情影响而中断的全球和地区产业链、供应链也难以完整修复。因此，"环球同此凉热"断已不是"诗和远方"，而是当下人类"同呼吸，共命运"的生活现实。

最后，此次疫情深刻揭示了全球公共卫生安全治理体系的弱点和短板。作为其基础，各国自身的公共服务水平和制度建设，尤其是治理理念、供给能力、协调效能等均显不适。作为其内涵与机能，各国之间合作动力、规范和对公共物品投入保障与共享机制还远未得到充分、健全的发展。如果说"人类的每一次重大进步都是危机推动的"，那么新冠肺炎疫情正在为各国提供携手共建全球公共卫生安全共同体的难得机遇。

严酷的全球疫情和艰巨的防疫斗争也进一步昭示我们，"偏安一隅""以邻为壑"都是幻想和不现实的选择，单边主义、"一国优先"的思想已经落后于时代发展的潮流，而"人类命运共同体"理念的先进性、普适性则得到极大的强化，其重大理论和现实意义正在进一步彰显。

第一，21世纪人类生存图景已经发生重大转换，信息化、智能化技术的日益普及不仅将极大地改变人类生产活动的范式，也将促进各国社会之间全方位的对接与联系，从而更加激发马克思、恩格斯所预见的"个人获得全面发展其才能"共同体建设的动力。这是不以人的意志为转移的历史大趋势，也是检验新时代国家建设和国际关系发展的最新标准。执政者必须清醒认识和主动顺应这一趋势，其对外政策要超越"以权力为中心"旧观念、旧思维和旧路径，代之"以人民为中心"的新型世界发展观、国际安全观和全球秩序思想。新者，恰是适应各国人民不断变化、日益增长的发展需求而问世，也必将随着各国人民动员起来所产生的巨大联动效应，有力地冲击抱残守缺的"部落思维"和"国家中心主义"的营垒，代表着历史前进的最终方向。

第二，21世纪的人类发展不仅展现出更新的生产力和更高层次的开放格局，而且也提出调整和建立与之相适应的共同身份及生产关系的使命要求。"人类命运共同体"理念的精要之处，就在于它超越了民族、国家利益的传统视域，将一国的发展置于与其他国家相互依存、休戚与共的本质上加以考量，寻求"互利共赢"而非"零和博弈"。它具有更强的时代感和地域覆盖性，既符合全球生产分工体系日益精细化、扁平化的实际，也代表了各国人民密切的利益关联以及由此产生的共同身份。由此，"我们"将具有更广泛的代表性和不断弱化的排他性，不同文明、体制和发展环境所造成的国家特性会获得更多的正视与尊重，基于"非我族类"陈腐心态的传统安全观将被新型合作安全观所取代。显而易见，"人类命运共同体"较此前任何国际政治身份都更具进步意义，不仅为各国共同参与应对当下全球治理难题和安全挑战提供了更鲜明的正当性，也准确地标示出国际关系民主化的时代趋向。

第三，影响人类发展的任何思想都必须具有鲜明的实践指导意义，否则就会成为建构在沙滩上的楼阁，经不起现实的检验。21 世纪过去了 20 年，经济全球化急速推进造成日益明显的国际发展失衡，"治理赤字""信任赤字""和平赤字""发展赤字"四大矛盾集中爆发。要有效缓解和最终改进全球发展失衡问题，根本的出路仍在于合作。新时代的全球合作必须具有更加明确的"普惠、包容、共进"的导向，不应也不能回到"亲资本"和"重商主义"的老路上去。"人类命运共同体"理念强调各国经济和社会发展的相互协作，探索用"政策沟通、设施联通、贸易畅通、资金融通、民心相通"作为实践路径，形成"开放、协商、共建、共享"的新型国际合作范式，进而达到"在发展中解决发展赤字，通过合作减少信任赤字，以实实在在的和平红利来消除贫困等动乱的根源"。"人类命运共同体"理念还特别注重将"绿色、可持续发展"作为新型国际合作要义，强调人与自然之间的共生关系，不仅对各国研发新技术开发新产业、节省地球资源、转变生活方式等具有理论指导意义，也对进一步关照欠发达国家、小国、岛国的生存发展和安全利益具有现实感召作用。

作为新思想、新实践，"人类命运共同体"要真正变成"放之四海而皆准"的价值原则和行为规范，还需经过漫长的演进过程，必须完成几个方面的建设。

首先，习近平主席提出，"和平、发展、公平、正义、民主、自由是全人类的共同价值"。要通过"一带一路"等一系列实验性开放合作项目的外溢效应，促进共同利益的生成与认知，增加人类共同价值的实际存在感，使后者逐渐成为凝聚"人类命运共同体"的精神圭臬。

其次，要顺应新型全球化进程的客观需要，把握和利用好发展失衡和贫富差距持续加大、气候变化、地区动乱和大规模难民潮等紧迫安全挑战所蕴含的转机，在多边合作观念和方式上不断创新，推动未来全球"发展"与"治理"两大议题呈"双轮驱动"、并行不悖之势。

最后，"人类命运共同体"的建设重心在于打通民意，获得公众的理解和支持。在高度信息化的时代，任何重大国际合作的民意基础都至关重要。国家、企业等国际行为主体不仅需要更好地投入公共外交和履行社会责任，也要积极联合其他社会行为体组成有效的知识传播复合体，致力于将跨境合作所累积的利益、共识转化为新的常识与社会风尚。

译文：

Anti-pandemic Cooperation Reveals the Only Way to the Construction of a Community with a Shared Future for Mankind

Wu Baiyi[*]

"After a period of time, history creates a watershed". The COVID-

* Wu Baiyi, Senior Researcher, Former General Director of Institute of European Studies, Chinese Academy of Social Sciences, CASS.

19 pandemic pierced through the natural and man-made boundaries on the planet, posing an unprecedented grave challenge to the health and safety of mankind. It is a harsh, historic test. As the combat against coronavirus outbreak goes deep in various countries, the answers will be closer to the true nature of the times. They will also become the consensus motivating us to traverse the watershed and move towards post-pandemic common development.

First of all, against the background of a highly globalized economy, humans have considerably greater freedom of mobility and migration than the last century. Consequently, the capital chain, industrial chain, supply chain, information chain, and even interpersonal relationship chain have been formed and densely distributed across the globe. On the one hand, they are the objective reason for the spread of coronavirus. On the other hand, as they disintegrate national boundaries and resolve differences in income and power, all parties share the identity of victims, fighters, and winners. As Director-General Tedros Adhanom pointed out in his speech at the 73rd World Health Assembly, "It (COVID-19) has also reminded us that for all our differences, we are one human race, and we are stronger together."

Secondly, since the fight against the coronavirus was started around the world, all countries have supported each other by sharing data and information, experience in diagnosis and treatment, and health emergency supplies. Scientists, business people, and social organizations have also carried out conversations about the development of vaccines and related drugs. All this reflects human conscience and rationality in the face of a catastrophe. So far, there is no end in sight to the battle. Different countries have different peaks of the coronavirus, so any country that has emerged from the crisis before others cannot fully restore its economic and social life alone. Besides, it is difficult to completely repair the interrupted global and regional industrial chains and supply chains. Therefore, it has become a reality that humans around the world are now "sharing the same breath and destiny".

Thirdly, COVID-19 has profoundly exposed the weaknesses in the governance of global public health security. As the basis of global public health security, the public service and institution building of each country, especially the governance philosophy, supply capacity, and coordination efficiency, are not competent. As its connotation and mechanism, the driving force and norms for cooperation between different countries and the guarantee and sharing mechanism of public goods investment are far from fully developed. If we say that "every major progress of mankind is driven by a crisis", then COVID-19 is providing a rare opportunity for all countries to jointly build a global community of public health security.

The harsh coronavirus situation and the arduous fight against COVID-19 further reveal that the "drawbridge up" and "beggar-thy-neighbor" policies are pipe dreams and unrealistic choices. The ideas of unilateralism and "one country first" have fallen behind the trend of the times while the advanced, universal concept of "a Community with a Shared Future for Mankind" has been greatly consolidated, with its theoretical and practical significance being further demonstrated.

First, the 21st century has witnessed momentous changes in the prospects of human survival. The increasingly widespread application of IT and AI will not only transform the ways of production but also promote the all-round connection between various societies, thus stimulating the power to construct the Community that, according to Marx and Engels, enables "the all-round development of the individual". This is a historical trend that "does not depend on the subjective will of men" and the latest standard to test national construction and the development of international relations in the new era. All country leaders must have a clearly-headed grasp of the trend and actively adapt to it. In terms of external policies, the old mentality and old path of "revolving around power" must be replaced by the new "people-centered" view of world development, international security, and global order. This new concept comes out at an opportune moment to meet the ever-changing and growing development needs of people across the globe. It will definitely gather huge momentum as people worldwide stand together, assaulting the conservative camp of "tribal thinking" and "state-centrism" and representing the ultimate direction of historical progress.

Second, in the 21st century, new productive forces have emerged and the world is more open than before. Meanwhile, it is important to establish and adjust common identity and production relations corresponding with human development. The essence of the Community vision lies in that it transcends the traditional notions of national and national interests and seeks "mutual benefits and win-win results" instead of "zero-sum game", as it considers the development of a country within the context of the interdependence of nations. In step with the times and applicable to most parts of the globe, it satisfies the demands for the increasingly refined and flattened global division of production and stands for the close connection of interests of people of all countries and the resulting common identity. Therefore, "we" will have wider representativeness, with increasingly weakened exclusiveness. The national characteristics derived from different civilizations, systems, and development environments will gain greater respect. In contrast, the traditional security concept based on the old mentality of "alienating nations with different ideologies" will be replaced by the new concept of cooperative security. Obviously, the "Community with a Shared Future for Mankind" is more progressive than any previous international political identity since it not only provides distinct legitimacy for countries to cope with the global governance problems and security challenges but also accurately marks the trend in the democratization of international relations.

Third, any idea that shapes human development must be practical; otherwise, it is just a castle in the air. In the past 20 years, the rapid advancement of economic globalization has caused a distinct imbalance in international development, as exemplified by four major contradictions, namely, "governance deficit" "trust deficit" "peace deficit" and "development deficit". To effectively alleviate and ultimately redress the imbalance of global development, cooperation is still the only solution. Global cooperation in the new era must explicitly demonstrate "inclusiveness and common progress". We should not and cannot head back to the old "pro-capital" and "mercantilist" path. The notion of "a Community with a Shared Future for Mankind" emphasizes the economic and social cooperation between countries and explores the practical path of "policy communication, infrastructure connectivity, trade connectivity, financial integration, and people-to-people connectivity. By forming a new international cooperation paradigm of 'openness, extensive consultation, joint contribution, and shared benefits', it aims to eliminate the development deficit through development, reduce the trust deficit through cooperation, and eradicate the root causes of unrest such as poverty with real peace dividends". The concept also pays special attention to "green and sustainable development" and regards it as the essence of new international cooperation, with an emphasis on the symbiotic relationship between man and nature. This will not only provide theoretical guidance for countries to develop new technologies and industries, save the earth's resources, and improve people's lifestyles but also attract attention to the survival and security interests of underdeveloped countries, small countries, and island countries.

To turn this new idea and new practice into a "universally applicable" principle and code of conduct, there is still a long way to go and efforts must be made in the following fields:

First, President Xi Jinping puts forward that "peace, development, fairness, justice, democracy, and freedom are the common values of mankind". The spillover effect of a series of experimental projects based on open cooperation, such as the Belt and Road Initiative will help with the formation and perception of common interests and strengthen the presence of common values which will gradually become the spiritual paradigm of the Community with a Shared Future for Mankind.

Secondly, we need to follow the trends in new globalization and seize and make good use of the opportunities behind urgent security challenges such as unbalanced development, widening gap between the rich and the poor, climate change, regional unrest, and large-scale refugee movement. By constantly innovating the concept and model of multilateral cooperation, we can ensure that the two major issues of global "development" and "governance" will develop side by side.

Finally, the construction of the Community focuses on gaining public understanding and support. In a developed information age, popular will plays an essential role in any major international cooperation. Countries, enterprises, and other international actors need to invest more in public diplomacy and fulfill their social responsibilities. Moreover, they should work with other social actors to disseminate knowledge effectively and devote themselves to transforming the accumulated interests and consensus of cross-border cooperation into new common sense and social mainstream.

对人类共同命运意识的一次集体唤醒

王灵桂*

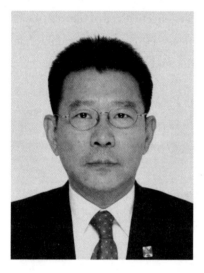

新冠肺炎疫情是波及所有人的人类悲剧。但在全球各国人民共同抗击疫情的生存之战中，人类命运与共的思想光辉，正以其强大的生命力和感召力，穿过疫情阴霾，照亮了人类未来发展之路，新的人类共同价值观呼之欲出。

2020 年伊始，在新冠肺炎疫情暴发后，许多国家（地区）和组织及时向中国伸出了援手：雪中送炭捐助物资、发表声明道义支持、网友发帖鼓劲打气。在中国疫情得到基本控制后，中国政府投桃报李，迅速向相关国家（地区）和国际组织捐赠物资、派遣专家、分享数据、交流经验。疫情无情，人间有爱，中国人民和世界人民共同谱写了彰显人类命运共同体的抗疫新篇章。

病毒肆虐，疫情凶险，唯有全球合作才能渡过难关。疫情感染和致死人数还在节节攀升，引发了全球极度焦虑和担忧。联合国秘书长古特雷斯表示，新冠肺炎疫情是联合国成立以来，人类面临的最大考验，呼吁国际社会加强团结，共同应对疫情。

此次共同抗疫是对人类共同命运意识的一次集体唤醒。面对凶猛

---

* 王灵桂，中国社会科学院副院长、国家高端智库理事会副理事长、研究员。

而至、不断蔓延的疫情，我们看到，全球科技工作者携手合作、共享数据和信息。中国科学家将病毒基因组排序迅速与世界各国分享、不同国家科技工作者共同加紧研制药物和疫苗；我们看到，世界各国守望相助，互赠抗疫物资，有的国家把自己最后的库存抗疫物资毫无保留地捐赠出来；我们看到，许多国家明智地摒弃体制机制和意识形态争论，以高度的国际人道主义精神，和国际社会一道，面对人类的共同敌人病毒。凡此种种，均说明人类命运共同体不是口号，而是丰富、生动的实践。

人类命运共同体理念开始进入国际关系实践层面。从疫情暴发至今，全球各国在探索之中，走过了形式多样、政策迥异、效果不同的抗疫之路。但是，全球已经达成了一个基本共识：疫情肆虐无国界，任何国家和任何人都难独善其身，唯有以保护人类未来和人民福祉为出发点，走团结合作的命运共同体之路，才是制服新冠肺炎疫情的唯一正确选择。2020 年 3 月 26 日召开的 G20 领导人应对新冠病毒肺炎特别峰会，就是这个共识的里程碑式象征。从一定意义上说，给各国人民生命安全和身体健康带来巨大威胁的疫情，正在催生新的国际价值观。在新的国际价值观中，人类命运共同体意识将成为其主要理念。

人类命运共同体理念代表着人类的进步。实事求是地看，新冠肺炎疫情并非人类首次面临的集体威胁，如鼠疫曾经让欧洲沉寂多年，西班牙大流感曾按下了世界前进的暂停键，等等。在诸如此类的灾难浩劫来临时，很多人将其当作难以抵挡和抗拒的超自然现象。但是，今天，世界已经在全球化进程中大大进步，人类已经形成了空前紧密的命运共同体关系。美国学者托马斯·弗里德曼评论说："每个国家和个人，不分民族和肤色，不论贫穷和富有，都是受害者，新冠病毒已成为全人类名副其实的共同敌人。"面对全人类的共同敌人，世界各国团结起来战胜病毒的可能性已成现实，各国寻求合作抗疫也成为应有的政策选项。这将是人类历史上以命运共同体意识共克时艰、共抗风险的开端，标志着人类共同价值观的巨大飞跃和进步。正如习近平主席在 G20 特别峰会上强调指出的："重大传染性疾病是全人类的敌人。新冠肺炎疫情正在全球蔓延，给人民生命安全和身体健康带来巨大威胁，给全球公共卫生安全带来巨大挑战，形势令人担忧"，"只要我们同舟共济、守望相助，就一定能够彻底战胜疫情，迎来人类发展更加美好的明天"。

人类追求命运共同体努力的道路依然崎岖。任何一种美好的愿望和价值理念，并不会天然形成，更不会自然诞生。在疫情不断蔓延的情况下，人类命运共同体理念正在越来越深入人心，正在不断彰显其巨大世界意义和全球价值。国际社会齐心协力、团结合作，共同汇聚起战胜疫情的强大合力，携手赢得这场危及人类安全和未来的斗争，这一趋势已成共识。但是，我们也不得不指出，在这种大势之下，某些人逆势而行，或罔顾生命、漠然视之；或玩忽职守、应对不力；或心存侥幸、朝令夕改；或将疫情政治化，捞取政治得分和选票；或抗疫不力而推卸责任、甩锅他国。

人类新的共同价值之光，正崭露于中国人民和世界人民团结合作抗疫的丰富实践中。全球200多个国家和地区、70多亿人口，我们因何而紧密相连？未来又将走向何方？基于对历史和现实的深入思考，中国领导人给出了中国答案。从2013年年初到2018年年中，习近平主席在近70个不同的重大国内国际场合，深刻阐述了命运共同体这个宏大课题，展现了中国领导人面向未来的长远眼光、博大胸襟和历史担当。2018年3月11日，第十三届全国人民代表大会第一次会议通过的宪法修正案，将"推动构建人类命运共同体"正式写入了宪法序言。2017年1月18日，习近平主席在联合国日内瓦总部发表的《共同构建人类命运共同体》重要演讲，明确指出"宇宙只有一个地球，人类共有一个家园"，但是"人类也正处在一个挑战层出不穷、风险日益增多的时代。世界经济增长乏力，金融危机阴云不散，发展鸿沟日益突出，兵戎相见时有发生，冷战思维和强权政治阴魂不散，恐怖主义、难民危机、重大传染性疾病、气候变化等非传统安全威胁持续蔓延"。在包括重大传染性疾病在内的严峻挑战面前，让和平的薪火代代相传、让发展的动力源源不断、让文明的光芒熠熠生辉，既是各国人民的期待，也是各国政治家应有的担当。

大道至简，实干为要。中国和世界各国团结合作抗疫的实践说明，构建人类命运共同体，打造人类新的共同价值观，关键在于行动。同时，也再次验证了"建设一个普遍安全的世界"的极端重要性，因为"邻居出了问题，不能光想着扎好自家篱笆，而应该去帮一把"。在这次伟大的抗疫斗争中，中国人民已经走出了坚实的一步。在这场伟大的抗疫斗争中，那些自私者、狭隘者、搅局者、甩锅者，都应反思并回到正确的人类发展道路上来，共筑人类新共同价值观的基础。

中国是负责任的国家，中华民族是信守承诺的民族。我们相信，中国促进世界共同发展的决心不会改变，中国携手世界打赢人类抗疫之战的愿望不会改变。

译文：

A Collective Awakening of the Awareness of Shared Future for Mankind

Wang Linggui[*]

COVID-19 is a tragedy affecting all humankind. However, in the global battle against the coronavirus, the light of a Community with a Shared Future for Mankind has pierced through the haze of COVID-19 and illuminated the road to future development. A new set of common values is about to emerge.

Following the coronavirus outbreak at the beginning of 2020, many countries (regions) and organizations immediately extended a helping hand to China by delivering medical supplies, issuing statements of support, and

* Wang Linggui, Senior Research Fellow, Vice President of CASS, Vice Chairman of Board of Directors, National Top Think Tank Council, Chinese Academy of Social Sciences.

posting encouraging messages online. After the coronavirus was basically under control, the Chinese government repaid their kindness by swiftly donating supplies, sending experts, sharing data, and exchanging experience. In the face of a merciless pandemic, the Chinese people and the people of the world have written a new chapter in the battle that demonstrates the Community with a Shared Future for Mankind.

Only global cooperation can we overcome the grave situation. The increase in the number of confirmed cases and deaths is still rising has greatly alarmed the world. Recently, UN Secretary-General Antonio Guterres said that "COVID-19 is the greatest test that we have faced together since the formation of the United Nations," calling for solidarity in the international community to tackle the crisis.

This joint anti-epidemic campaign is a collective awakening of the awareness of a Shared Future for Mankind. Facing the ongoing, fierce pandemic, we can see that scientists around the world work together to share data and information. Chinese scientists share the viral genome with countries around the world promptly. Scientists from different countries work together to develop medicines and vaccines. Various countries offer each other medical supplies, and some even donate the last stock of their supplies without reservation. Many countries have wisely set aside institutional and ideological disputes and fought against COVID-19, the common enemy of mankind, with an international humanitarian spirit. All these show that the Community with a Shared Future for Mankind is not a slogan but a rich, vivid practice.

This concept has entered the practical level of international relations. Since the coronavirus outbreak, countries all over the world have fought battles of various forms and with different policies and different outcomes. However, the world has formed a basic consensus: since the pandemic respects no borders, it is difficult for any country or anyone to stay safe; only by putting the future of mankind and people's wellbeing first and building a Community with a Shared Future for Mankind featured by solidarity and cooperation can we overcome the COVID-19 pandemic. The G20 Extraordinary Leaders' Summit on COVID-19 held on March 26 is a milestone symbol of such consensus. In a sense, while posing a great threat to life and health, the pandemic is creating new international values. In the new international values, the main idea of which is the Community with a Shared Future for Mankind.

The concept of a Community with a Shared Future for Mankind represents the progress of mankind. In fact, COVID-19 is not the first threat to mankind. For example, the bubonic plague once devastated Europe and the 1918 influenza pandemic brought world development to a halt. When such disasters loomed, many people regarded them as irresistible supernatural phenomena. However, with remarkable progress in globalization, the world has become an unprecedented close community with a shared future. American scholar Thomas L. Friedman said, "Every country and individual, regardless of nationality and color, whether poor or rich, is a victim to the coronavirus, which has become a real common enemy of mankind". As it is realistic for the world to act as one to defeat the virus, cooperation should become a proper policy option for all countries. This will be the first time that humans have ever surmounted difficulties with the awareness that the world is a community with a shared future. It marks significant progress in common values. As President Xi Jinping emphasized at the Extraordinary G20 Leaders, Summit: "Major infectious disease is the enemy of all. As we speak, the COVID-19 outbreak is spreading worldwide, posing enormous threat to life and health and bringing formidable challenge to global public health security. The situation is disturbing and unsettling." "But through solidarity and mutual assistance, we will prevail over this outbreak and we all will embrace a brighter future for mankind."

The road to the Community with a Shared Future for Mankind is still full of twists and turns. Any kind of good wishes and values do not come into being naturally. With the continuous spread of the virus, the concept of the Community with a Shared Future for Mankind is being widely accepted, with its global significance and value constantly being demonstrated. It has become a consensus that the international community should work together to win the battle against the coronavirus and protect the security and future of humanity. However, it should be pointed out that some politicians dismiss this general trend or even go against the trend, treating life with indifference, or fail to fulfill their duty and respond to the pandemic effectively; or change policies frequently, or politicize the pandemic to score political points and secure votes, or shirk responsibility and shift the blame onto other countries because of their poor anti-coronavirus performance.

The light of new common values is coming out of the rich, practical cooperation on the fight against COVID-19 between the Chinese people and the people of the world. Why are we, more than 7 billion people in over 200 countries and regions, closely connected? What does the future hold? Pondering on both history and reality, Chinese leaders have provided the Chinese answers. From the beginning of 2013 to mid-2018, President Xi Jinping had expounded the Community with a Shared Future for Mankind on nearly 70 different domestic and international occasions, displaying his long-term vision, broad mind, and historical responsibility. On March 11, 2018, with the amendment to the Constitution being adopted at the first session of the 13th National People's Congress, "promoting the construction of a Community with a Shared Future for Mankind" was enshrined in the preamble of the Constitution. On January 18, 2017, President Xi Jinping delivered an important speech entitled "Work Together to Build a Community of Shared Future for Mankind" at the United Nations Office at Geneva, in which he clearly pointed out that "There is only one Earth in the universe and we mankind have only one homeland. Mankind is in an era of numerous challenges and increasing risks. Global growth is sluggish, the impact of the financial crisis lingers on and the development gap is widening. Armed conflicts occur from time to time. Cold War mentality and power politics still exist. Non-conventional security threats, particularly terrorism, refugee crises, major communicable diseases, and climate change, are spreading. " In the face of grave challenges, including major infectious diseases, let's pass on the torch of peace from generation to generation, sustain development and ensure civilization flourishes: This is what people of all countries long for; it is also the responsibility that states persons of our generation ought to shoulder.

A great vision, simple and pure, requires credible actions. The practice of cooperation between China and other countries in fighting the pandemic shows that actions hold the key to the building of a Community with a Shared Future for Mankind and the creation of new common values. At the same time, it has once again verified the extreme importance of "building a universally safe world", because "When neighbors are in trouble, instead of tightening his own fences, one should extend a helping hand to them." In this historic battle, the Chinese people have taken a solid step forward. In this historic battle, those who are selfish and narrow-minded and those who spoil the anti-pandemic progress and pass the buck should introspect about their behavior and return to the right track of development to jointly build the foundation of new common values.

China is a responsible country, and the Chinese nation is a nation that keeps its promises. We are confident that China's determination to promote the common development of the world will never change, and its desire to join hands with the world to win the battle against COVID-19 will never change.

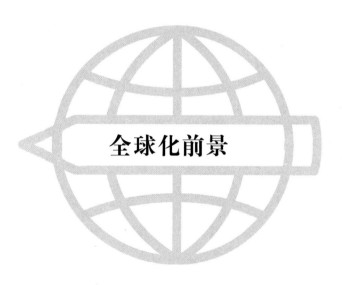

全球化前景

全球化趋势不可逆转之际的"大流行"

格列格尔茨·W. 科洛多科（Grzegorz W. Kolodko）[*]

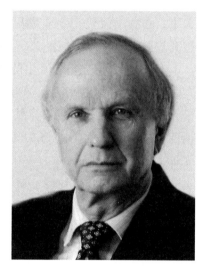

新型冠状病毒大流行给世界投下了巨大的阴影。它使人类面临难以置信的挑战，这些挑战与其他消极的大趋势以及尚未解决的经济、社会和政治问题同时出现。上一次国际金融和经济危机的系统性和结构性根源并未消除。新自由主义——意识形态、政治和错误地以牺牲多数人的利益来让少数人致富的规则——使全球化不能更加包容、如中国人所说的"双赢"。此外，自然环境的破坏和全球变暖的进程并没有停止。收入不平等仍在加剧。人口结构的失衡加剧，导致大规模移民。由于无法以协调一致的方式解决日益严重的跨国问题以及缺乏对相互依存的全球经济进行管理的机制，政治紧张局势正在加剧。伴随着美国对中俄两国挑起的贸易摩擦，仇外主义、沙文主义、新民族主义和保护主义的"幽灵"正在抬头。

前景黯淡

从西亚北非政治动荡到"黑人的命很重要"，从"占领伦敦"到

---

* 格列格尔茨·W. 科洛多科，波兰前副总理。

63

"占领华尔街"，从德里到圣地亚哥，从法国到阿尔及利亚，人们纷纷走上街头举行抗议。将会有更多的抗议和示威，混乱也会加剧。世界需要的是新思想和伟大的领导者，具有全球视野的政治家，而不是高喊"美国优先"的煽动者！为了避免破坏世界文化和经济的无政府主义，我们需要新的思想和发展理念，如新实用主义。

我们正在经历一个匪夷所思的时代，在这个时代，一个十几岁的瑞典少女竟然比美国总统更聪明、更有责任感；在这个时代，引领全球经济持续发展的希望寄托于中国和印度，而不是美国和日本；在这个时代，许多政客为更美好的未来而祈祷，因为他们无法创造美好的未来；在这个时代，企业家更乐于储蓄，而不是投资；在这个时代，愚蠢战胜智慧，侵害战胜共情。所有这些都是我们人类的功绩。

现代文明和经济全球化的这些大趋势同时发生，极为不利，而"大流行"之祸此时暴发，雪上加霜。没有人知道它到底什么时候会来，会是什么样子，但它显然终将到来。我在《真相、谬误与谎言：动荡世界中的政治与经济》（*Truth，Errors and Lies：Politics and Economics in a Volatile World*）一书中曾写到，我们正面临"大规模疾病、迅速蔓延的流行病、对身心具有破坏性影响的许多难民危机带来的日益严重的威胁"，"假定不会出现具有像艾滋病毒或'非典'那样致命潜力的新病毒，将是极为天真的，迟早会出现这样的新病毒"，而"在当今世界，面对流行病学威胁，越来越需要在治疗和预防政策上进行全球协调"。我写下这些话并不是有显著的洞察力，也不是一种悲观主义。

当森林被烧毁的时候，不是为玫瑰感到遗憾的时候。同样，现在不是对生产衰退感到遗憾的时候，因为这是人类为生存而斗争的时候。由于采取了激进而代价高昂的预防和治疗措施，数以百万计的人们的生命和健康得以被拯救，这比一些经济体势必遭遇的经济萧条造成的损失更有价值，毫无疑问，也比股票交易所损失的数万亿美元更有价值。股票的核心就是投机，因此也没什么可遗憾的，然而，养老基金价值的下降和流行病的经济后果不可低估——无论是在供求层面，还是在人类心理和社会意识层面，我们甚至在未来几十年后都将还能感受到其影响。

我们可以应对这些短期问题，尽管微观经济形势十分严峻，宏观经济后果也很严重。中国已经在其遵守纪律的社会和国家中控制住了局势，甚至表现得优于一些西方自由民主主义国家——这些国家也正在经历一场具有深远影响的根本性危机。

政府增加公共支出以支持经济复苏并保护有特殊需要的人群和个人是正确的。根据实际情况，需要注入数十亿，甚至数千亿美元。当然，对于大多数国家，这将增加预算赤字，在许多国家，将很难控制公共债务，但在目前的情况下，这样做是两害相权取其轻。许多国家的央行降低利率也是正确的。整个银行业都面临着巨大的挑战，它们必须通过相关措施来支持企业的金融流动性，特别是推迟偿还贷款，并将贷款分期发放给受危机影响的企业。

长期影响更为重要。毫无疑问，由生产和消费动荡引起的"大流行"将影响到跨国公司的做法和经济政治家对参与外国生产和供应链的态度。我认为，当最坏的情况过去后，理智将占上风，全球化不仅不会受到损害，恰恰相反，它将变得更为双赢。然而，在这种情况发生之前，反全球化的愤恨将占上风。

艰难时期

可怕的是恐惧和非理性主义、狭隘主义和民族主义、特殊主义和保护主义的抬头。我们不仅受到看不见的东西——微观的新型冠状病毒——的威胁，而且还受到肉眼所见的东西的威胁：仇恨。种族仇恨、伊斯兰恐惧症、中国恐惧症、俄罗斯恐惧症，缅甸佛教徒对罗兴亚人的态度，伊朗什叶派对阿拉伯半岛逊尼派的态度，保守的英国人对来自布鲁塞尔的欧洲人的态度，排外的法国人对中东移民的态度，对陌生人和其他非本地人的厌恶，对来自"烂国家"的人们和那些"墨西哥的强奸犯"的厌恶，对那些同性恋和异教徒的厌恶。

当唐纳德·特朗普从区域自由贸易协定中脱身，转而反对为防止全球变暖而战的《巴黎协定》、关于伊朗核计划的安排、与俄罗斯关于控制中程导弹系统的协定、世界贸易组织的特权时，这对和平合作和包容性全球化进程造成损害。中国领导人是对的，多边主义，而不是单边主义必须成为全球经济和政治博弈的准则。

"大流行病"后，应通过逐步过渡到一种新的实用主义的方式来创造一个更美好的未来，这种新的实用主义是一种旨在实现经济、社会和生态三重平衡的经济学理论和发展战略，这样人类才有机会拥有共同的未来。(毛悦校译)

原文：

Pandemic at the Time of Irreversible Globalization

Grzegorz W. Kolodko [*]

The COVID-19 pandemic lays a long shadow on the world. It puts humanity in the face of incredible challenges that coincide with other negative mega-trends and unresolved economic, social and political problems. The systemic and structural sources of the previous global financial and economic crisis have not been removed. Neoliberalism-ideology, politics and wrong regulation enriching the few at the costs of many-prevents globalization from being more inclusive, win-win, as the Chinese say. The processes of devastation of natural environment and global warming has not been stopped. The growth of income inequalities continues. The demographic imbalance is deepening enforcing a mass migration. Political tensions are growing due to the inability to conciliatory solve the growing transnational problems and the lack of mechanisms to govern the interdependent global econo-

[*] Grzegorz Witold Kolodko, Former Deputy Prime Minister, Poland.

my. The ghosts of xenophobia and chauvinism, new nationalism and protectionism are rising, accompanied by trade friction provoked by the United States to China and Russia.

Doom and Gloom

People take to the streets from the "political conflicts in West Asia and North Africa" to the "Black Lives Matter", from "Occupy London" to "Occupy Wall Street", from Delhi to Santiago, from France to Algeria. There will be more protests and demonstration and chaos can increase. The world needs new ideas and great leaders, global statesmen, not demagogues shouting America First! In order to avoid anarchization, which would devastate culture and economy all over the world, new ideas and development concepts are needed, such as new pragmatism.

We are experiencing bizarre times when a Swedish teenager is smarter and more responsible than the American president; when hopes for keeping the global economy on the development path are placed in China and India, not in the USA and Japan; when many politicians pray for the better future because they are unable to control its creation; when entrepreneurs prefer to save rather than invest; when stupidity triumphs over wisdom and aggression over empathy. It is all our human merit.

Here is the scourge of pandemic joined the extremely unfavorable coincidence of these mega-trends of modern civilization and the globalized economy. Nobody knew when exactly it would come or what it would look like, but it was obvious that it would come. This is not clairvoyance—or rather gloom—mongering—when I wrote in *Truth, Errors and Lies: Politics and Economics in a Volatile World* that we are facing "a growing threat of mass diseases, fast-spreading epidemics, the many refugee crises with their destructive physical and psychological effects" that "it would be the height of naive to assume that there will be no new diseases with the lethal potential of HIV-AIDS or SARS. It has to happen sooner or later" and that "In the contemporary world, there is an increasing need for the global coordination of treatment and prevention policies in the face of the epidemiological threat. "

It is not time to regret the roses when the forests are burning. It is not the time to regret the decline in production as it is the result of the struggle for human life. Millions of those whose, due to radical and costly preventive and curative measures, lives and health are saved, are much more valuable than losses caused by the recession, which some economies will not miss, and no doubt than those trillions lost on stock exchanges. Its speculative core is nothing to regret, however, the decline in the value of pension funds and the economic consequences of a pandemic cannot be underestimated—neither those on the supply and demand side, nor those in the sphere of human psyche and social awareness, what we will be felt even after the next decades.

We can handle these short-term issues, although there are plenty of dramatic microeconomic situations, and their macroeconomic consequences are also severe. China, within its disciplined society, has mastered the situation. Even better than some states of liberal democracy, which is also undergoing a fundamental crisis with far-reaching consequences.

Governments are right increasing public expenditure to support economic recovery and to protect populations and individuals in special need. Depending on the realities, there need to be sensibly pumped billions, hundreds of billions of dollars into the economy. Of course, in most countries this will increase the budget deficit, but in these circumstances it is a lesser evil, although in many countries it will be difficult to keep public debt in check. Central banks of many countries are also right to lower interest rates. The entire banking sector faced a huge challenge, which must use its arsenal of instruments supporting the financial liquidity of enterprises, especially by postponing loan repayments and their distribution in installments to companies hit by the crisis.

Longer-term consequences are more important. Undoubtedly, pandemics caused by turbulences in production and consumption will have their mark on the approach of transnational corporations and on the attitude of economic politicians to becoming involved in foreign production and supply chains. I think that when the worst is over, sanity will prevail and globalization will not be harmed, quite the opposite—it will indeed be more win-win type. However, before this happens, anti-globalization resentments will prevail.

Tough Times

What is to be feared is the rise of phobia and irrationalism, parochialism and nationalism, particularism and protectionism. We are threatened not only by what cannot be seen—the microscopic coronavirus—but also by what can be seen with the naked eye: hatred. Racial hatred, Islamophobia, Sinophobia; Russophobia; Buddhists from Myanmar to Rohingya, Shiites from Iran to Sunnis from the Arabian Peninsula, conservative English to Europeans from Brussels; xenophobic French to Middle East immigrants. Aversion to strangers, to others, not from here; those from "shithole countries" and those "rapists from Mexico"; those colorful and these infidels.

It harms peaceful cooperation and inclusive globalization when Donald Trump disengage in regional free trade agreements, turns against the Paris Agreement on combating global warming, an arrangement on Iran's nuclear program, an agreement on controlling the medium-range missile system with Russia, the prerogatives of the World Trade Organization, the WTO. The China's leaders are right that not unilateralism, but multilateralism must be the principle of the global economic and political game.

In the post-pandemic world a better future should be created by a gradual transition to a new pragmatism—an outlay of economics theory and development strategy aiming at triple balance: economic, social, and ecological. Then there will be a chance for a shared future for mankind.

孤立主义无市场

鲁卡·马里安·斯卡兰提诺
（Luca Maria Andrea Scarantino）[*]

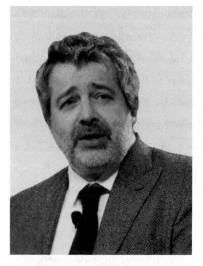

窗外，位于米兰市古老中心的街道看起来冷冷清清。与全球千百万人一样，我们处于完全封城之下。在这样一个初春时节，在这样一个忙碌的日子里，我们从未经历过这样一份寂静。望向窗外已成为一种催眠式体验。每隔一刻钟左右，我们会瞥见远处经过的某个行人。我们听到的唯一的城市噪音是附近大街上循环往复的空荡荡的电车，以及疾驰而过的救护车。

我和老伴都明白，几周来，我们与全世界亿万人口拥有共同的命运：宅在家里。这种情况从来没有发生过，我们得学会适应它。最初几周里，我们的工作重心是制定一份可以接受的日程表。作为学者，我们相对幸运一些。虽然限足在家，我们每天仍然能够阅读写作，与其他城市和国家的同行通信。然而，在封城一再延长带来的最初恐惧逐渐消退后，我们得以对新"常态"生活进行反思。我们忽然意识到，隔离未必是我们最初惧怕的一种孤独状态。当数亿人同时身涉其中时，社会疏离就成为一种唤醒人类共同体意识的共同体验。自疫情大流行以来，我们与亲友及各地同行之间交流的短信、视频电话和聊天彰显了共同的感

知和情感：无论身处湖北、新泽西、伦巴第、巴黎还是阿根廷，我们都带着同样的惊异生活在当下的状态之中。我们此刻的目光比以往的"常态"生活时期更加一致。

诸多迹象表明，非同凡响的事情正在发生。大自然正以一种不为我们熟悉的方式在城市中苏醒。青草从欧洲古老城市的石缝间冒出；鲜花在广场上绽放；野猪、野鸭、野鹿甚至野狼在寂静和清新氛围的吸引下踱入市区。除了环境的明显改善外，我们也感知到内心的变化。在围绕疫情的无数分析、探讨、数据和评论之外，似乎萌发了一种强大的人类共同体意识。未来几年，我们将清晰地回忆起这段隔离的日子，并把它用作与他人打招呼的共同代码。"对了，你在新冠肺炎疫情期间怎么样啊？"在指代一种集体体验时，这类问题很可能会成为我们对话的常见内容，即便我们与对方互不相识，或者相隔万里。

在很大程度上，这可能是一种存在主义的危机应对方法，但它有助于我们想象社会互动和全球互动将会受到怎样的影响。几乎毫无例外地，民众和国家领导人都将愈发感知到世界的现实关联性。较之宏观经济、文化和环境问题，健康危机更可能导致我们看待外部世界方式的深刻改变。简言之，人们越来越相信，地球另一边发生的事情与我们有着直接的关联。如果我们把危机看作是一个了解其他文明的机会，而不是一个强化现有偏见与成见的借口，那么我们可以从这场危机中学到很多。或许，对病毒的恐惧将有助于我们更好地理解世界文化和社会的复杂性。

疫情还给我们的观念带来了另外一个重要变化：人们变得更富有群体意识，这是社交距离产生的副产品之一。数亿人宅在家里，真真切切地感受到了前所未有的团结感。但我们也开始以一种不同的方式来看待自己的生活方式。社会隔离现象在人类历史上曾屡见不鲜。几千年来，人类社会面临流行病、侵略、瘟疫、劫掠和破坏的威胁。今天，很多地方仍然处于这些威胁之下。疫情也为我们提供了一个反思人类历史地位的机会。现在看似非同凡响的事情是我们祖先的日常体验；但我们已经忘记，我们的生活方式既不是坚不可摧的，也不是不可避免的。现代性使我们自诩为人类史上的特权存在，而此次疫情则是一个强烈的提醒：我们不是！

可以预见，疫情将促使人类转变对全球性问题的看法，如气候变化、人类健康、社会不平等。我们对地球的关爱（现在已经是一项重要的国际日程）可能会受到疫情引发的新的情感效应的驱动。当我们呼吁孩子们（包括那些在消费社会的温室中成长起来的孩子们）减少废弃物，以免对世界上的其他孩子产生不必要的影响时，他们可能会比我们更深切地体会到这一呼吁的意义。

这是否意味着国际合作将变得更加顺畅、更加没有争议？可能不会。但疫情也暴露出了另一个怪象：孤立主义（作为政治立场）的虚无性。任何国家、民族或帝国都不能假装自己孤立于其他国家、民族或帝国的行为之外；任何国家、民族或帝国都不能假装自己的行为不会影响到其他国家、民族或帝国。虽然我们不期望疫后的现实政策会发生重大改变，但我们至少可以在短期内做出现实的预测：我们将更加清楚地认识到，我们的日常和社会行为将散播到世界各地，并具有全球性影响。我们将更乐于承认我们的生活方式不再是可持续的。

我们在过去几周所作的努力（接受继续宅在家里），还可能会使我们对日常习惯的改变不再抵触。也许不经意间，我们会发现自己能够欣然放弃新冠肺炎疫情发生前那些不可或缺的行为。我们甚至可能意识到，世界各地、不同文化和不同文明的人类都抱有同样的感受。（王文娥翻译）

原文：

Isolationism Has No Market

Luca Maria Andrea Scarantino[*]

The streets under our windows, in the ancient heart of Milan, look de-

---

* Luca Maria Andrea Scarantino, President, International Federation of Philosophical Societies.

serted. As millions of other people, we are under total lockdown. We can hardly recall a comparable quietness, especially during such a busy time as the early weeks of spring. Looking out of our window has become a hypnotic experience. Maybe once every fifteen minutes, someone can be spotted walking in the distance. Meanwhile, the only city noise we can hear is that of empty tramways circulating along the nearby boulevard, and of ambulances running across town.

My spouse and I are well aware that for weeks now we have been sharing the same fate as hundreds of millions of humans across the world. Stay home. This was obviously an unprecedented circumstance, to which we had to learn how to adjust. In the first weeks, our main concern was to set up an acceptable daily routine. As scholars, we are relatively lucky. Confined inside our home, we can still spend our days reading, writing, and corresponding with colleagues in other cities and countries. As the initial scare slowly wore off with the repeated extensions of the lockdown, however, we were able to somewhat allow ourselves to reflect on our new state of "normal" life. We felt, unexpectedly, that isolation may not necessarily be such a lonely condition as we originally feared. We realized that social distancing, when practiced by billions of individuals at the same time, becomes a shared experience, for it triggers a feeling of shared humanhood. The hundreds of messages, video calls, and chats that we exchanged with relatives, friends, and colleagues across the world since the beginning of the pandemic show a span of common feelings and emotions: whether in Hubei, New Jersey, Lombardy, Paris, or Argentina, we live our current condition with the same astonishment. Our gazes are much more uniform now than they have ever been in our previous "normal" life.

There are obvious signs that something extraordinary is going on. Our cities show marks of an unfamiliar awakening of nature. Grass is growing through the cracks between the cobblestones of our old European cities; flowers bloom on the squares; wild boars, ducks, deer, even wolves are now entering city areas, heartened by the new silence and by the lack of human smell. Aside this visible transformation of the environment, though, we can feel that something inside our minds is also changing. Alongside countless analyses, talks, data, and comments on all things surrounding the pandemic, a powerful sense of common humanity seems to be born out of this experience. For years to come, we will vividly recall this time of isolation, and use it as a common code to relate to people we will meet. "So, what about you during the COVID-19 pandemic?" —knowing that it refers to a collective experience, this kind of question may well become a recurrent part of our conversations, even if we are fully stranger to our interlocutors and live thousands of miles apart.

This may be a rather existential approach to the crisis, and nonetheless it may help us imagine how our social and global interactions could be affected. Citizens and country leaders are, with few exceptions, becoming more sensitive to the actual relatedness of our world. More persuasively than macroeconomic, cultural, or environmental concerns, health emergencies might prompt a far-reaching change in the way we look at the outer world. To put it plainly, it has become increasingly difficult to believe that something that is happening on the other side of the world does not directly concern us. We might learn a lot from this crisis, if we took it as an opportunity to increase our understanding of other civilizations, rather than as just another pretext to enhance existing prejudices and stereotypes. Perhaps, the fear of the virus will help us become more deeply acquainted with the cultural and social complexity of our world.

Yet another significant change in our mindset might occur as an effect of the pandemic. An increased sense of togetherness could stem out of it as a byproduct of the ongoing social distancing. Billions of humans, closed in their own homes, do sense what we could see as an increased feeling of solidarity. But we may as well start looking at our own lifestyles in a different way. Social isolation has been a recurrent phenomenon in human history. Societies have faced pandemics, invasions, plagues, pillages, and devastations for millennia. In many areas of the world, they still do. This pandemic also gives us a chance to reflect on our place in history. What now seems so extraordinary to us was a frequent experience for our ancestors; but we have forgotten that our way of life is neither indestructible nor inevitable. While modernity taught us to think of ourselves as privileged beings in the course of human history, this is a violent reminder that we are not.

Foreseeably, issues of global import, such as climate change, health concerns, and social inequalities, would eventually be viewed differently. Our care for the planet, already a key topic in international agenda, is likely to receive a new push by the emotional effects of the pandemic. When our children, including those who were raised in the typical comfort of a consumerist society, are told to reduce waste, as this may have unwanted effects on other children across the world, they may sense the meaning of this request much more intensely than we ever did.

Does this mean that international cooperation will become smoother and more uncontroversial? Probably not. But it is another oddity of this pandemic to reveal the vanity of isolationism as a political stance. No country, nation, or empire can pretend to be immune from the consequences of others' actions; and none of them can any longer pretend that its actions do not affect others. Although we should not expect actual policies to change dramatically as an effect of the pandemic, at least in the short run, we can realistically predict that an increased awareness of the global effect of our daily and social behaviors will spread across the world. We are becoming less reluctant to admit that our ways of life are no longer sustainable.

The effort we made in the last weeks, accepting to be confined at home for an extended period of time, might also erode our resistance to change our daily habits. Perhaps without noticing it yet, we may discover soon that we can happily give up behaviors that we considered indispensable before the COVID-19. We may even realize that such sentiment is shared by fellow humans across the planet, cultures, and civilizations.

疫情之后：全球化走弱还是走强？

柏钗·丹维瓦塔 （Pornchai Danvivathana）

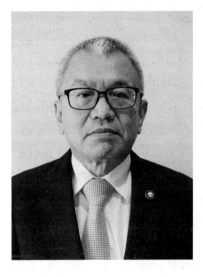

当新型冠状病毒来袭时，没有任何一个国家做好准备。病毒迅速蔓延至世界各地，目前全球仅有不到十个国家未受病毒感染。为控制病毒传播，多国政府被迫宣布进入紧急状态，或对他国或城市实行包括禁飞在内的封锁。截至目前，很多企业和行业仍处于无限期关闭或暂停经营的状态上。此时此刻，人们才意识到疫情大流行已对各行各业造成的冲击有多么的严重。

当下困难时期，各国政府和企业已感同身受地明白疫情给日常活动带来的种种干扰和破坏。不可否认的是，新型冠状病毒的全球传播其实也是全球化的一种结果。目前人们对全球化进程走势看法不一，本文认为，疫情之后，全球化进程不仅不会衰退，而且会在 5G 电信网络普及之后得到进一步强化。

全球化已在路上

尽管存在种种反全球化的不满情绪，特别是 1999 年世界贸易组

＊ 柏钗·丹维瓦塔，亚洲合作对话（ACD）秘书长。

织（WTO）在西雅图举行部长级会议的时候表现得更为突出，但是在过去的三十年里，全球化依然赢得了广泛支持。通常情况下，人们将关注的重点放在全球化对贸易和经济的影响上。诸多研究表明，全球化将带来包括国内生产总值（GDP）在内的经济福利的增加，也助力区域间和区域内互联互通的实现。另外，5G 技术的发展将使人们享有更强大的网络空间，物联网（IOT）用户数量的不断增长也在加速全球化进程。

诺贝尔奖获得者约瑟夫·斯蒂格利茨（Joseph E. Stiglitz）在其著作《重新审视全球化及其不满》中解释到，唯有改革，才能使全球化惠及世界并迈向更加公平的世界。不过，我认为，当前的物联网和人工智能（AI）的快速发展，正在进一步刺激商品、服务和人员跨境流动的快速增长，全球化进程也因此得以持续下去。

当前，发达国家和发展中国家正在为第四次工业革命做准备，而作为第四次工业革命的核心——数字技术仍有赖于对高质量互联网基础设施和网络的投资，以支持 5G 技术的应用。唯其如此，全球化才有可能得到进一步加强。

现今某些国家的商业中断有可能被新型冠状病毒继续拖延下去，而那些未受疫情影响的国家正努力维持正常运行，以对抗新型冠状病毒来袭。从新型冠状病毒的发现到被确诊为具有传染性，再到全球大流行，仅仅用了几个月的时间，且该病毒有 14 天的潜伏期，之后才能被迅速诊断。在疫苗得到开发之前，无人可以担保尚未被波及的国家是不是会被感染。

截至目前，国际社会已达成了一个非正式共识，即解决疫情的关键是保持社交距离或进行物理隔离，更不用说要尽可能佩戴口罩和经常使用洗手液。人们被要求居家办公，并被鼓励通过视频会议进行业务往来，否则疫情很容易失控，使人们陷入被感染的危险境地。

有趣的是，不管社区是否实行宵禁，当人们被要求待在家里或保持物理隔离时，人们对生活方式的改变如网上购物，有着普遍的适应能力。正因此，送货上门也获得更多的市场份额。

现在看来，即使流行病得到控制，商店也不会再像以往开门营业，人们也不会再像以往乘坐日常的交通工具赶去上班了。疫情使人们更加确信，借助电子商务等技术，也可以生存得更好。由于数字技术像全球化一样无国界，许多工作场所可能会更加依赖数字技术，以取代人力。实际上，上述行为在疫情期间已得到印证。最重要的是，各国政府和私营部门已认识到，全球化和互联互通在很大程度上已助力各国，特别是发展中国家从世界各个角落获取信息，从而使他们面临更加公平的竞争环境。相应地，人们也意识到，在线上交易和自动化日益盛行的今天，人工智能和数字经济必将节省大量工时和生产成本。

结论与前景

即使今后疫情得到了有效控制，各国仍有可能继续推进数字经济的发展。根据国际货币基金组织（IMF）2020 年 4 月发布的《世界经济展望报告》，由于全球大流行导致多国采取部分或全面封锁、关闭工作场所以及禁飞等举措，全球经济正面临有史以来最为严重的衰退。国际货币基金组织还呼吁加强多边合作，共享设施和专业知识，并敦促全球共同努力，分享治疗方法和待开发的疫苗技术。

控制跨国传染需要国际合作，唯有这样，才能确保疫情得到完全遏制，并助力恢复全球的企业经营和人们的日常生活秩序。基于此，亚洲合作对话（ACD）愿意为加强 35 个成员国开展国际合作提供平台，以解决类似流行病和自然灾害带来的难题。当前有关抗疫的经验和教训，将成为下届部长级会议讨论的主要议题。不管怎么说，合作抗疫在当下任何时候起步都为时不晚。

目前，我们还不能自以为是地去恢复日常营业，毕竟我们需要为将来的任何大流行做好更充分的准备。为此，我们不仅应进一步加强合作，动员包括亚洲经验和最佳实践在内的各种资源，以改善公共卫生保健体系，还应评估储备物资是否或在多大程度上能够做到全天候待命。最重要的是，面对日益加强的全球化进程，唯有做出适当改变才是当下可行的出路。（冯北京翻译）

原文：

After the Pandemic, Will Globalization Fade or Intensify?

Pornchai Danvivathana[*]

Introduction

When the COVID-19 broke out and became epidemic, no country in the world was well prepared at that time. The contagion rapidly spread through all regions of the world and left fewer than ten countries unaffected by the epidemics. It warranted governments of many countries to announce the state of emergency or impose lockdowns on their countries or cities, including flight banning, in order to control the pandemic widespread. It appears that until now lockdowns are still applicable, thus businesses and industries have to close down or suspend their operations indefinitely. At this point in time, people around the world realize how severe the impact of the pandemic has caused on people from all walks of life.

During the difficult time, governments and commercial businesses are aware of the disruption of their operations at all levels. Of course, the global widespread of COVID-19 is a result of globalization which connects people to people and countries to countries. Nevertheless, when the situation subsides, globalization may or may not change its course. However, it won't fade, but intensify, especially until after 5G telecommunications network is available.

---

* Pornchai Danvivathana, Secretary-General, Asia Cooperation Dialogue.

Part Ⅰ of this article introduces the idea that globalization will continue its course and could be intensified when 5G is in place. Part Ⅱ shows that globalization had been given popularity, but at times it witnessed discontent, particularly in developing countries. Part Ⅲ offers recommendations and prospects related to globalization.

Globalization Will Take Its Course

Globalization has gained its support over the past three decades, even though there have been some sentiments against globalization, particularly when the World Trade Organization (WTO) held its Ministerial Meeting in Seattle in 1999. In most cases, focus was put on the impact of globalization on trade and economy. A lot of studies have identified that globalization would increase a lot of economic benefits, including gross domestic product (GDP). It also boosted connectivity at both the inter-regional and intra-regional levels. Moreover, the development of 5G technology will allow people in all regions to have access to powerful wireless capacity. The growing number of users of the Internet of Things (IoT) will help accelerate the impact of globalization.

Joseph E. Stiglitz, a Nobel Prize winner, explained in his book, titled *Globalization and Its Discontent Revisited* that globalization needs to be reformed for a fairer and better one. To me, globalization will take its course because IoT and artificial intelligence (AI) will stimulate fast-growing cross-border flows of goods, services and people despite some advantages and disadvantages of globalization.

As the developed and developing countries are preparing themselves for the Fourth Industrial Revolution, the digital technologies which are at the heart of the Fourth Industrial Revolution need to promote investment in high-quality internet infrastructure and networking that would support the application of 5G technology in a proper fashion. Therefore, it is likely that globalization will be intensified.

80

The disruption of business, caused by COVID-19, may be prolonged in some countries. Yet such non-affected countries are currently struggling to, at least, maintain the status quo of their health care to fight the coronavirus. It took only several months for the coronavirus to become a global pandemic after it was known as an infectious disease. This disease could not be rapidly detected until after the incubation period of fourteen days is over. Until after a vaccine to cure this disease is available, there is no guarantee that those countries will never become infected.

It appears that the international community has reached its informal consensus that social distancing or physical isolation is key to resolve the pandemic, let alone the common recommendation on wearing face masks and application of hand sanitizer as often as possible. Those who are at work are required to work from home and doing business via video-conferencing is widely encouraged. Otherwise, employers and employees could easily be put at risk while the outbreak goes beyond control.

It is interesting to note that people are adaptive or resilient by changing their lifestyle to online shopping while they need to stay at home and observe physical distancing, regardless of whether curfews are enforced in their communities. That is the reason why door-to-door delivery business has gained more market shares compared to others in the services sector.

It seems that, after the coronavirus pandemic is kept under control, it may not be business as usual when shops are open and people may rush to work by means of their routine modes of transportation. Then, the pandemic has given everyone a good lesson that human being may survive with the best use of technology, like e-commerce. As digital technologies know no borders, as is the case for globalization, many workplaces may rely more on digital technologies to replace the dominance of human workforce. This is, in fact, a matter of behavioral change, which has been practiced during the difficult time at many workplaces. On top of that, governments and the private sector have realized how much the impact of globalization and connectedness have help countries, particularly developing countries, to access information from every corner of the world so that their level playing-field is improved. In this context, all would realize how AI and digital economy would save a lot of manhour and costs of production, including time consumption, when online transactions and automation are increasingly available at hand.

Conclusion and Prospects

It is likely that countries tend to promote the digital economy, even after the widespread of COVID-19 is kept under control. According to the IMF's World Economic Outlook in April 2020, the global economy will face the worst ever recession due to partial or comprehensive lockdowns and closures of workplaces and flight banning in many countries, as a result of the global pandemic. The IMF also called for multilateral cooperation in sharing equipment and expertise to fight against COVID-19. It continued to urge a global effort so that therapies and vaccines, if developed, could be accessed.

It becomes vivid that this transnational contagion requires international cooperation to ensure its complete containment and to break disruption of businesses and the livelihood of people in every continent, who have been spending their lives at home over a monthly-long period.

Along this line of thinking, the Asia Cooperation Dialogue (ACD) is another forum for strengthening the international cooperation among thirty-five Member States to arrive at a resolve to handle such pandemics and natural disasters in the future. The experience gained throughout this difficult time and lessons learnt so far regarding COVID-19 treatment could be an agenda item for discussion at the next ministerial meeting. It is never too late to sit down together and aim at any concrete action in a concerted effort to wipe out COVID-19 and other disasters.

In no case should we allow complacency to lead us to revert to business as usual since we need to be better prepared for any future pandemics. In this regard, not only that we should collaborate further on how to mobilize resources, including experiences, as well as best practices, in Asia to improve public health care system, but also on whether or to what extent stand-by arrangements of stockpiles of tools and equipment could be reviewed for their 24/7 availability. On top of that, adaptive behavioral change is inevitable while globalization is intensifying.

全球化的前景

翁诗杰（Ong Tee Keat）*

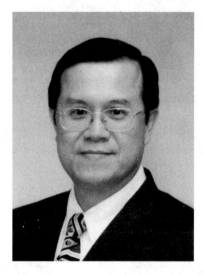

在过去的三十年里，全球化已经成为推动世界大部分地区经济发展的催化剂，对发展中经济体尤为如此。与此同时，全球化也见证了以多边主义为前提的全球治理新模式的出现。自此，世界进入了全方位快速变革的范式转变时代。

多边主义已被视为解决全球关切议题的可行办法，并也一直在协调国际社会在应对若干全球危机中发挥作用。近年来的成功实例，包括应对2008年国际金融危机，以及协调国际社会共同应对埃博拉病毒、中东呼吸综合征等流行传染病。

然而，随着经济全球化大幅度重塑了全球经济格局，它也因此似乎成为全球化备受瞩目的焦点。经济全球化以自由贸易之名拆除了保护性关税壁垒，并史无前例地让经济领域的供需双方分别对接到广大的全球市场和供应链，这些特点备受赞誉。我们从未想过跨境的互联互通能达到这种广度和深度。发展中经济体是经济全球化的主要受益者。该机制的成功也再次提高了国际合作的可行性。其实，早在第二次世界大战后，随着联合国及其附属机构的成立，国际合作的基础即已奠定。

---

* 翁诗杰，马来西亚新亚洲战略研究中心主席。

　　然而另一方面，经济全球化借以依托的经济联通性与自由度在欠发达的经济体当中却仍有争议。经济全球化备受指责的缺陷是，它加剧了贫富国家之间日益扩大的经济差距。弱国认为全球化市场并不是他们所期许的公平竞争环境。事实上，由西方大国决定的游戏规则，并不曾为弱小国家的愿景留下任何的空间。在这些国家容易获取的工业生产材料和劳动力供应链，乃至他们给商贸、服务所提供的现成市场，往往只沦为增添强国财富的工具而已。

　　当这场永无休止的辩论仍在持续之际，新型冠状病毒的暴发已给全球化带来了一次大考验，同时也催使国际社会必须采取协调一致的应对措施。但不幸的是，美国竟背弃了众望所盼，缺席了领导全球抗击流行病的斗争，这是史无前例的，同时也让全球化的国际合作备受阻挠。

　　美国特朗普总统所谓"美国第一"的夸夸其谈，已清楚表明他会牺牲多边主义全球化来推动单边主义的意图。新冠肺炎疫情暴发前，美国退出应对全球气候变化的《巴黎协定》和联合国教科文组织的举动，已清楚表明他执意反对国际合作的立场。最近正当美国的新冠肺炎疫情扩散至高峰时，特朗普宣布冻结美国对世卫组织的资金援助，这一举动再次印证了他的立场。

　　相反的，中国迅速向疫情严重的国家派遣医疗队，并提供物资的行动，与西方对新型冠状病毒的不力应对，形成了鲜明的对比。遗憾的是，中国善意的人道主义援助，却被刻意描绘和夸大为旨在扩大中国地缘政治影响力的宣传手段。与美国相比，中国疫情的死亡率相对较低，这项初传的捷报惹恼了华盛顿，只因它令美国霸权的自豪感受损。所谓北京捏造疫情的死亡率和发病率数据——这类毫无根据指控的出现，自然也就成为意料中事。同时，中国抗疫经验的分享，也被语无伦次地喻为"输出中国模式"的特洛伊木马。而拒绝从非英语国家人民的惨痛经验中吸取教训的习性，似乎也已成为西方必然的傲慢。友爱精神已抛掷窗外，这大大损害了国际的合作和团结。

　　这引发了对全球化现有模式的有效性重新审视的思潮。在全球一些民粹主义政客的鼓吹下，披上民族主义外衣的单边主义正不断升级，我们明显更需要对此思考。

　　必须承认的是，这次百年一遇的疫情是检测国际合作和团结的试金石。单边民族主义不太可能在疫情后就此消失。目前全球经济前景总体呈现悲观严峻态势，人们普遍认为新冠肺炎疫情之后的全球化，势将面临最大的考验。当今世界正处于十字路口。值此人类可能面临越来越多的生存挑战之际，与全球合作相对立的民族主义和单边主义，只会让世界以更快的速度毁灭。新型冠状病毒的肆虐只是一个警钟，提醒我们，在灾难面前，人类命运相同，只有通过集体的智慧和团结，我们才可能生存下来。

国际社会必须重塑全球化的现有模式，以免为时已晚。迫切的生存威胁与抗灾救援的问题，理应更受到重视。重塑的全球化应该超越经济领域，并且必须从过去的不足吸取教训，让新阶段的全球化摆脱任何霸权主义国家的控制。国际合作机构也必须被赋予足够的资源，让其能够履行职责，以建立一个没有政治干预的共生模式。

总而言之，只要常理能够克服短视的民族主义诉求，全球化的前景仍将保持乐观。人类应该拥抱这希望的召唤，以全球化 2.0 之名赋予这一重塑模式新的生命。（董方源翻译）

原文：

Prospects of Globalisation

Ong Tee Keat[*]

In the past three decades, globalisation has been a proven catalyst for economic development in vast parts of the world, notably in the developing economies. In parallel, it has witnessed the emergence of a new model of global governance premised on multilateralism. The world has since been

---

* Ong Tee Keat, Chairman, Centre for New Inclusive Asia, Malaysia.

thrusted into an era of paradigm shift fraught with rapid transformation in all dimensions.

Multilateralism, having been cherished by the world as a viable model of addressing global concerns, has so far been instrumental in coordinating international response in handling several crises. The successful handling of the financial crisis in 2008 and the coordinated international responses to such pandemic outbreaks as Ebola and MERS-CoV, to cite a few, are among which, the most recent testimonies of multilateral globalisation.

Nonetheless, economic globalisation seems to have taken the centre stage as it has enormously reshaped the global economic landscape. Having been characterised with an unprecedented wide access to the supply chains and market worldwide, it has generally been greeted with effusive accolades for tearing down the protective tariff barriers in the name of free trade. Never before have we ever dreamt of trans-border connectivity being brought into fruition to such length and breadth. The developing economies stand out to be the main beneficiaries of economic globalisation. The success stories of its mechanism further increase the viability of international cooperation, of which the foundation was well laid after WWII with the inception of the United Nations and its affiliated agencies.

While, on the other hand, the economic connectivity and liberty that it was underpinned upon remain contested in the less developed economies. Economic globalisation is flawed for having contributed to an ever widening gulf of economic disparity between the rich and the poor nations. The disadvantaged claimed that the globalised market after all is not a level playing field as they anticipated. Ground rules of the game, dictated by the Western powers, have virtually left no room for the aspirations of the small and weak nations. Both the easy access to material and labour supply chains for industrial production as well as ready market for goods and services in these countries is generally perceived as a boon enriching only the rich and powerful.

While this endless debate rages on, the COVID-19 outbreak has put the globalisation to test, prompting the dire need for coordinated and coherent international response. But this was unfortunately thwarted by the unprecedented absence of the United States in leading a global fight against the pandemic which was widely expected.

President Trump's bombast of "America First" is a clear manifestation of his agenda of promoting unilateralism at the expense of multilateral globalisation. His action in withdrawing from the Paris Agreement in climate change and the UNESCO prior to the coronavirus outbreak was a clear sign of his implacable objection to international cooperation. His recent announcement of freezing the US monetary support for WHO amid the height of coronavirus spread in his own country further speaks volumes of his stance.

On the contrary, the immediate dispatch of medical team and supplies to the wantonly pandemic-stricken countries by China stands out starkly in contrast with the botched handling of COVID-19 in the West. Unfortunately the well-intentioned Chinese humanitarian aid was deliberately portrayed and blown out of proportion as a propaganda move designed to expand the geopolitical influence of China. The preliminary success story of China in fighting the contagion by keeping a low fatality tally vis-a-vis that of the US has riled Washington as the latter's hegemonic pride was perceived to have been bruised. Unfounded allegations against Beijing of fudging statistics of outbreak fatality and morbidity seem to be par for the course. Experience sharing in fighting the outbreak by the Chinese was incoherently labeled as a proverbial Trojan Horse for exporting the Chinese model. Refusal to learn from the bitter experience waded through by the non-anglophone people appears proudly endemic among the West. Spirit of camaraderie is thrown out of window much to the detriment of international cooperation and solidarity.

This has triggered provoking thoughts of revisiting the efficacy of the prevailing globalisation model. Such need grows even more pronounced in the wake of escalating unilateralism shrouded with nationalism that was trumpeted by some populist-centric politicians across the globe.

While acknowledging that the once-in-a-century outbreak is a real litmus test for international cooperation and solidarity, the spectre of unilateral nationalism is unlikely to vanish after the outbreak. Currently the global economic outlook appears pessimistically grim across the board. The post-COVID-19 years ahead are widely believed to be even more challenging for globalisation. The world is now at the crossroad. While more potential existential challenges for mankind are looming, nationalistic unilateralism antithetical to global collaboration would only doom the world to apocalyptic devastation at a faster pace. The ravaging coronavirus is merely a wake-up call to dawn upon us that we have a shared destiny in face of calamities which we could only probably survive through concerted wisdom and solidarity.

This warrants the necessity for the international community to reinvent the current model of globalisation before it is too late. Greater emphasis should be attached to the pressing issues of existential exigencies and disaster response to reshape the present model into one that goes beyond economic collaboration.

Parallel to this, drawing from the past experience of shortfalls, the new phase of globalisation must be free from the stranglehold of any hegemon's dictate. International institutions for global collaboration must be empowered with sufficient resources to discharge their duties in favour of forging a symbiotic model, bereft of political intervention.

All in all, the prognosis of globalisation would remain optimistic so long as common sense prevails over myopic nationalistic appeals. Mankind should seek to embrace this beaconing hope by giving the reinvented model a new lease of life in the name of Globalisation 2. 0.

疫情后的世界格局：
全球化放缓，还是加快？

黄 平[*]

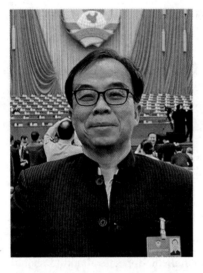

2020 年注定要载入世界历史史册。

现在，各国还在与新型冠状病毒搏斗中，我们还是无法预知病毒蔓延什么时候会结束，或者哪怕暂告一段落，疫情以后的世界还会是过去那个世界吗？

即使病毒蔓延以前，我们也见证了世界多极化、恐怖主义、全球气候变化、华尔街金融风暴、各种形式的民粹主义和保护主义、难民危机、逆全球化……

可以说，我们的确正在见证着百年未有之大变局。这时，不确定性本身成了最大的确定性，风险、危机、"陷阱"、"黑天鹅"，随处可见；社会失范，政治失序，制度失灵，安全失控，精英失职，在西方国家已不是个别现象；国际关系重组，国际规则重写，国际秩序重建，国际格局重构，是正在或将要发生的事情，不论人们愿意不愿意。

更突如其来且让人难以置信的是，这本来就已经充满了不确定性

黄平，香港中国学术研究院常务副院长、研究员。

的百年未有之世界大变局，进入 2020 年居然又平添一大变数：新型冠状病毒的全球性蔓延，给所有的国家及其公共卫生与防疫体系都来了个措手不及。

到目前为止，世界卫生组织或别的权威机构还不能明确告诉人们究竟这病毒从何而来？将持续多久？下一步会蔓延到哪里？哪些人更易感染或更可能会轻症转重症？究竟什么时候能研发出并广泛投入使用针对它的有效疫苗？

只要这些问题医学上还没明确答案，各国的体制机制上也并不都清楚如何妥善应对，抗疫，就仍然必须是第一位的。至于它带来了经济停摆、社交暂缓、"自由"受限、旅游不再、餐饮萧条、失业加重，恐怕就都只能是不得不面对的两难境地，因为，说到底，前者直接关系到的，是生还是死，而后者所涉及的，更多是快还是慢、多还是少。

而且，由于迄今我们所知所熟所能用到的国际层面的制度、机制、组织，更多的是第二次世界大战结束后为了防止人类再度陷入战争，也为了在和平基本能维护的环境下谋求经济社会发展，而几乎很少（例如世界卫生组织）有主要是为了预防和制止病毒大流行大蔓延而设计的，连这方面的专业人员、预算经费、组织架构、体制机制也都极端薄弱，在有的国家还几乎是形同虚设。这为有效抗疫又增添了难度。

概括起来，是否可以这样说：

第一，这次疫情暴发，所有人和国家、政府、组织、机构，谁也没有先见之明，没有谁提前就知道它将要暴发，更没有谁提前就知道如何妥善应对它，故根本没有任何根据去无端猜忌别人一开始没有采取更高明的措施，更没有资格去事后诸葛亮般地指责别人为什么没有做得更好。

第二，这次病毒降临，对所有人和国家、政府、组织、机构，都是一次大考，能经受住考验的，不是某种抽象的概念、制度，而是实际的应急与组织动员能力，尤其是面临紧急的公共卫生危机时的应急能力和治理能力，其中包含（但不限于）：国家的组织力、民众的配合度，社区的管理水平、个人的自觉行为，防疫体系的健全性与可行性、医护人员的专业水平与奉献精神，等等。

第三，这次疫情突发，谁也不能提前推论甚至断言哪个国家根本不可能在大考中取得好成绩，如果有好成绩就一定有诈。

第四，这次疫情蔓延，使本来就还没有从2007—2008年国际经济危机中完全恢复过来的各国经济变得更加低迷或进一步放缓，失业人数之多已经成了某些大国自从大萧条以来最为严重的经济社会问题，故也无法从原有版本的经济政策中直接找到解困之道，包括试图逆全球化而上，不仅要自我"优先"，而且不惜单方面"脱钩"。

第五，这次抗疫，对所有人、所有国家、所有政府、所有组织、所有机构，都是全新的挑战，它使本来就已经高度不确定的世界变得更加不确定，使我们本来就面临认识范式与治理方式转换的巨大压力变得更加沉重。

这个时候，世界各国需要的，不是危言耸听，但我们也要重视诸如"新冠肺炎疫情之后，世界将不再是原来的样子""新冠危机标志着一个转折点"之类的预言或警言，这会使我们更加冷静、现实、理性。

在这突如其来的病毒蔓延背后，我们面对的大问题是：在一个全新的挑战与危机、风险与机遇面前，我们，世界各国的人们，究竟要往哪里去、应该怎么去。

从时间序列上说，一开始，疫情不论发生在哪里、蔓延到哪里，人们的第一个"本能的"反应，都首先是自保，乃至于最先都会用"各自为战"的手段去应对。

而当自保不成时，或无法自保、不足以自保时，第二个（也是"心理的"）反应，其甚至可能还更糟，那就是：互相指责，互相推诿。当然，这其中也不乏政客试图通过"指责""推诿"来转移视线、转嫁矛盾，并推卸自己失职和无能。

因此，如果出现了下述情形，我们也不必大惊小怪：自己越是不能有效应对疫情，越是要指责别人，尤其是要无端指责那些比自己抗疫更有力也更有效，因此也得到更多关注的国家和社会。

这次这场世纪抗疫，现在还无法知道还将持续多久，或还将蔓延至何处，还会导致多少生命的付出、多少社会成本的损失，更不可能宣告何时方可取胜，而且，对我们所有人所有国家的大考还没有结束，一个更难的考题是：人类究竟能否在突如其来的大危机大灾难大瘟疫面前互相携手、共同抗疫？

人类，在一个越来越小，也部分地被旧式的发展与安全模式不断破坏的地球上，一方面地缘政治、权力纷争等仍然挥之不去，另一方面却可能掉进死胡同，落得个玉石俱焚。

进入21世纪以后，一者以资本、商品、服务、科技、信息和人员的大流动为特征的本轮全球化以超越西方世界原来所设想的广度和深度迅速发展，二者非西方国家和地区在这轮全球化中以几百年来从未有过的规模、速度和势头成为世界格局中的重要力量。在这种情况下，世界是继续按照事实上的丛林法则玩零和游戏，还是有可能走出一条不同的互鉴互补、合作共赢的道路？

如果没有这场大疫情，没有它的突如其来和如此蔓延，也许，很多人会对非零和非丛林的新秩序新格局继续怀疑或保留，哪怕口头上也会说"这也可以是一个好主意"，但内心仍认定无论是经济竞争还是政治博弈，都只能是你多我少、你输我赢，甚至是你死我活。

但是，人算不如天算。一场瘟疫天灾，让我们越来越看到了病毒是人类的共同敌人。没有共同敌人，人们就感觉不到彼此有共同利益；如果没有共同利益，也就谈不上共同责任；如果利益不分享、责任不共担，命运共同体就似乎离我们还太遥远。

当然，这里面必然内在地包含着艰难困苦，未知的不确定性中还会有荆棘丛生。如果没有哪怕仅仅是针对这一次全球性的非传统的公共卫生安全挑战而进行的艰苦努力，而继续走各自为战之路，不但口头上舆论上对人甩锅，而且仍然遵从丛林法则、信奉零和游戏，那么，就不只是病毒会持续蔓延，病死人数会持续攀升，各国的卫生体系会面临崩溃，正常的经济和社会生活无法恢复，而且，世界真的可能再度陷入大混乱、大萧条。

反过来说，我们面临的这次大疫大考，又使得人类命运共同体不再只是一个美好的愿景。由于病毒蔓延、病人剧增，在生还是死这个终极命题面前，人类迈向一个更开放、更公平、更可持续的全球化，并携手共建一个健康共同体、命运共同体，就成为现实的理性选择。

这么说来，"新冠将永远改变世界秩序"，而不是疫情之后又回归过去，至于它是促进了还是加快和改善了全球化，还要等时间来回答。

译文：

World Landscape after the Pandemic: Slowing or Accelerating Globalization?

Huang Ping[*]

2020 is destined to go down in history.

As the world is still fighting the virus, it is still impossible to predict when the pandemic will end or even temporarily come to an end. Some are wondering: will the world remain the same after COVID-19?

Even before the coronavirus, we had seen world multi-polarization, terrorism, global climate change, Wall Street financial crisis, various forms of populism and protectionism, refugee crisis, deglobalization ...

It can be said that we are indeed witnessing momentous changes unseen for a century. At this point, uncertainty itself becomes the greatest certainty. Risks, crises, "traps" and "black swans" are everywhere. Social anomie, political disorder, system malfunction, security out of control, and the elite's dereliction of duty are common in Western countries. Reorganization of international relations, rewriting of international rules, and reconstruction of international order and landscape are happening or going to happen, whether

---

* Huang Ping, Senior Researcher, Executive Vice President, Chinese Institute of Hong Kong.

we like it or not.

What is even more unexpected and unbelievable is that despite all these uncertainties, another one was added in 2020: the coronavirus pandemic has caught all countries and their public health and prevention systems unawares.

Up to now, the World Health Organization or other authorities have not been able to confirm the origin of the virus. How long will the pandemic last? Where will it go next? Who is more susceptible or more likely to turn from mild symptoms to severe symptoms? When will an effective vaccine against COVID-19 be developed and widely used?

As long as there are no clear medical answers to these questions and all countries do not know clearly what to do, fighting the pandemic must be the top priority. COVID-19 has led to the economic shutdown, suspension of socializing, restricted "freedom", stagnant tourism and catering business, and increased unemployment. We are hence faced with a dilemma of protecting life or reopening the economy.

Besides, the international systems, mechanisms, and organizations, which we have known and can turn to, are mostly used to prevent new wars after World War II and seek economic and social development in an environment where peace can be basically maintained. But few (if there is, such as the WHO) are chiefly designed to prevent and stop a pandemic, with a terribly weak network of professionals, budgets, organizations, and institutions. In some countries, such a network exists in name only. This makes it more difficult to fight the coronavirus effectively.

It seems that we can conclude as follows:

Firstly, no individual, state, government, organization, or institution had ever known in advance that COVID-19 was about to break out, let alone how to deal with it properly. Therefore, there is no reason to suspect others of failing to take effective measures at the very start, and no one is qualified to blame others for not doing better with hindsight.

Secondly, the COVID-19 outbreak is a harsh test for all individuals, countries, governments, organizations, and institutions. What is needed to withstand the test is not some abstract concepts or systems, but the actual emergency response and ability to mobilize. In particular, the ability to respond to and manage a public health crisis is extremely important, including but not limited to national organization, people's cooperation, community management level, conscious behavior, a sound and feasible epidemic prevention system, and professional, dedicated medical staff.

Thirdly, no one can infer or even assert in advance that no country could achieve such good results in the test, and if so, there must be some conspiracy.

Fourthly, the world economy, which has not fully recovered from the financial crisis of 2007—2008, will become depressed or sluggish. The large-scale unemployment has become the most serious socioeconomic of some major countries since the Great Depression, so it is impossible to directly find a solution from the original economic policies, including trying to go against globalization, which entails not only "putting themselves first" but also "unilateral decoupling".

Finally, COVID-19 is a brand-new challenge to all individuals, states, governments, organizations, and institutions. It makes the already highly uncertain world even more uncertain and increases the already enormous pressure of changing our cognitive paradigm and governance.

At this time, what countries around the world need is not alarmist remarks. Yet we should pay attention to some predictions or warnings such as "the world will never be the same after the coronavirus" and "the COVID-19 crisis could mark a turning point" because they will make us calm, realistic, and rational.

A serious issue behind the sudden COVID-19 outbreak is: where should we, people of all countries, go and how can we get there in the face of a brand-new challenge and crisis, risk and opportunity?

In a time sequence, no matter where an epidemic breaks out, people's first "instinctive" reaction is to protect themselves and even deal with it by "going in their own way".

When it fails or when self-protection is impossible or ineffective, the second (also "psychological") reaction may be even worse, that is, shifting blames onto others. Of course, there are many politicians who try to divert attention and shift contradictions by "passing the buck" to cover their dereliction of duty and incompetence.

Therefore, we need not feel surprised by the following situation: the more one fail to fight the pandemic effectively, the more one wants to put the blame on others, especially those countries and societies that are more powerful and effective in fighting the virus and therefore attract more attention.

At present, it is impossible to know how long it will last, where it will spread, how many lives will be claimed, and how many social costs will be incurred. It is even more unlikely to announce when we will win the battle. Besides, the harsh test for the world is not over yet. A more challenging question is: is it possible that all humans stand together and overcome the unexpected serious crisis?

Living on increasingly narrower earth partly damaged by the old path to development and security, humans still cling to geopolitical and power conflict, even at the risk of self-destruction.

In the 21st century, globalization has developed rapidly, which is characterized by the rapid flow of capital, goods, services, technology, information, and personnel. Both of its breadth and depth are beyond the original expectation of the West. Also, in this round of globalization, with scale, speed, and momentum unseen for hundreds of years, non-Western countries and regions have played a vital role in the global landscape. Under such circumstances, will the world continue to play the zero-sum game based on the de facto law of the jungle, or will it be possible to take a different path of mutual learning and win-win cooperation?

Without the sudden outbreak of COVID-19, many people may continue to have doubts or reservations about the new order that discards the zero-sum game and the law of the jungle, even if they say "this may be a good idea" but still believe that be it economic competition or political game, it is all about victory and defeat, life and death.

However, man proposes but God disposes. This quasi-natural calamity has made us more and more aware that coronavirus is the common enemy of mankind. Without a common enemy, people will not sense the common interests they share; without common interests, there will be no common responsibility; with no shared interests and duties, the Community with a Shared Future for Mankind seems far out of reach.

Of course, there must be hardships inside and there must be thorns in the unknown uncertainty. If we did not endeavor to address this non-traditional challenge to global public health security but continued to go in our own way, if we not only verbally shifted the blame onto others but also follow the law of the jungle and the zero-sum game, then the virus will continue to spread, claiming more lives, ravaging the health systems of various countries, and devastating normal economic and social life. Moreover, the world may slide into chaos and another Great Depression.

On the other hand, because of the test, the Community with a Shared Future for Mankind is no longer just a beautiful vision. Due to the spread of the coronavirus and the sharp increase in infection cases, the Community with a Shared Future for Mankind that embraces a more open, fairer, and more sustainable globalization has become a realistic, rational choice for human beings in the face of the life-and-death question.

In this sense, only time will tell whether the coronavirus pandemic promotes or improves globalization, which "will forever alter the world order" rather than keep the world as what it was.

全球化前景

王灵桂[*]

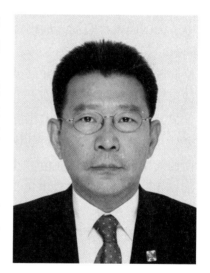

　　全球化的本质是思想、物质和生产的全球联通。在人类文明的绝大部分时间里，受制于交往手段，人们的全球化努力主要集中在邻近地区。随着火车、汽车、飞机的大规模商业使用，空间距离被大大压缩，真正意义上的全球化才开始出现。互联网的出现，又极大地助力全球化浪潮，进一步丰富和全球化的形式和内涵，全球之间的联系从来没有像今天这样如此便捷快捷。因此，现代科技的发展，是目前我们看到的全球化形成的基础和保障。从这个意义上讲，疫情从物理上隔绝人们之间的联系，只说对了一半。物质的联系受到阻隔，但是网络世界的联系，不但没有受到阻隔，而且得到了极大的发展。各种远程诊断、远程教学、云端会议和网上消费等得到急速发展，就是典型的例子。疫情期间全球化的这个特点，将会在疫后继续得到发展。因为人们突然发现，过去长途跋涉十几个小时旅途来开会的困扰，实际上通过网络视频完全可以瞬间解决。网络手段的极大丰富和多领域运用，将继续是疫后全球化的主要特征之一，但是全

---

　　[*] 王灵桂，中国社会科学院副院长、国家高端智库理事会副理事长、研究员。

球化对世界发展的意义并没有改变。原因在于：互相交往、互联互通是人类的本性，也是实现人类幸福的手段与途径。从古至今，这个特点从来没有改变过。唯一改变的，是人类的幸福指数越来越高。因此，疫情过后全球化不但不会停止，反而会以更加崭新的形式和更加丰富的内涵呈现并造福于全世界人民。

全球化作为世界各国人民追求幸福生活的不变途径，已经得到了人们的普遍认可。这是全球化的生命力之所在，更是其未来发展的原动力。但是，我们也不能不看到，很长一个时期以来，全球化到底还有没有前途的问题，已经引起了国际社会的普遍担忧。其中，美国因素是造成人们困扰的主要原因。作为世界上最大的发达国家，美国对外政策由全球扩张向孤立主义回调，坚持前者理念的建制派和主张后者的保守派分化日益严重；美国借口在国际社会维持领导者的治理成本不断上升，正在失去领导意愿，又不愿意别国发挥某种补充作用；随着国际新生力量的不断崛起，美国开始重新评估其构建的开放、多边的国际规则体系在保障其实现自身利益方面的效率，其政策取向由"全球模式"向半封闭乃至封闭的"俱乐部模式"转变；美国自由主义主导的世界秩序观和国际规范，强调美国样本的"普世性"，不承认基于大国实力的地缘政治逻辑，在某种程度上导致了美国与其他大国之间的矛盾和冲突；西方主流价值观遭遇质疑，西方社会分裂加剧，既体现在精英阶层内部的分化，也体现在保守力量与自由主义建制派的政策分歧，还体现在精英阶层与公众之间的认同分歧和矛盾。因此，一个时期以来国际社会普遍出现的所谓"逆全球化"担忧，实际上是美国政策犹疑和多变造成的不确定性。这个特征在当前抗击疫情的过程中，得到了淋漓尽致的体现。2020 年 5 月 29 日，美国总统特朗普召开记者招待会，对因疫情而死亡 10 余万人的困局、美警察虐杀黑人民众的血腥事实视而不见、只字不提，而一味执意坚持对中国指责、执意脱钩，就是典型的例证。从这个意义上说，疫后的全球化将不会再是美国一家独大，而是多种力量共商共建共赢的格局。

美国主导的全球化进程受阻与西方保守力量回调，将在各个领域影响国际秩序和国际规范。其中虽存在诸多变数和不确定性，但总体而言，中国的机遇大于挑战。在抗疫新冠病毒肺炎斗争中，中国政府的表现，国际社会有目共睹。抗疫的成绩单，说明美国作为领导者的道义制高点和软实力不复当年；在多边和全球治理层次上，美国不愿承担全球化和全球治理中的领导责任，为中国占据全球治理和自由贸易的道义制高点提供了机会；西方内部矛盾频发，美国内部斗争愈演愈烈，世界乱象需要中国这样的新生崛起力量进行适当平衡。

有两个消息能对我们预测未来全球化的基本图谱有所启示。2020年5月27日，德国总理默克尔公开发表演讲指出：由27个成员国组成的欧盟与中国的关系将成为其政府的重中之重，"我们欧洲人将需要承认中国在国际体系的现有结构中占据领先地位的决定性作用"，她还表示将与中国达成一项投资协定，并在应对气候变化和全球健康方面密切合作。5月30日，新加坡《联合早报》发表文章称，东盟十国和中国承诺致力维持开放市场、避免实行不必要的限制贸易措施。在此之前的29日，中国与东盟发表《中国—东盟经贸部长关于抗击新冠肺炎疫情加强自贸合作的联合声明》，重申将密切合作以对抗疫情，并呼吁共同减缓疫情对全球和区域贸易与投资的冲击；承诺迅速有效地分享抗疫信息和经验，"促进对抗新型冠状病毒药品和疫苗的生产和获取"，"展示东盟—中国面向和平与繁荣的战略伙伴关系精神"。5月23日，习近平总书记在全国"两会"期间看望政协会议经济界委员的讲话中，也再次强调："大力推进科技创新及其他各方面创新，加快推进数字经济、智能制造、生命健康、新材料等战略性新兴产业，形成更多新的增长点、增长极，着力打通生产、分配、流通、消费各个环节，逐步形成以国内大循环为主体、国内国际双循环相互促进的新发展格局，培育新形势下我国参与国际合作和竞争新优势。"默克尔总理代表欧盟的表态和东盟—中国贸易部长的联合声明，反映了三大经济体共同推动新一轮全球化的决心，描绘了未来全球化的多元图谱。习近平总书记的"两会"重要讲话，展示了中国坚持改革开放的巨大决心，给世界吃了定心丸。因此，未来多元发展、合作共赢的全球化前景一定会更加光明，一定会更好地造福世界人民。

译文:

Prospect of Globalization

Wang Linggui[*]

The essence of globalization is the global connection of ideas, materials, and production. Since civilization was, for the most part, restricted by the means of communication, the efforts to globalize are mainly concentrated in neighboring areas. With the large-scale commercial use of trains, automobiles, and airplanes, the spatial distance has been greatly shortened, giving rise to globalization in a real sense. The advent of the Internet not only gave a strong boost to globalization but also enriched its form and connotation, making global communication convenient and fast as never seen before. Therefore, the development of modern science and technology is the foundation and guarantee for the formation of globalization. In this sense, the remark that the pandemic physically isolates people from each other is only half right. While the physical connection has been restricted, the world of online connection has developed rapidly, as exemplified by the speedy development of various remote diagnosis, distance teaching, cloud conference, and online consumption. This feature of globalization will continue to develop after the pandemic. This is because people suddenly realize that the trouble of attending a meeting by traveling for more than ten hours in the past can be tackled instantly by online video-conferences. The widely applied, enriched

* Wang Linggui, Senior Research Fellow, Vice President of CASS, Vice Chairman of Board of Directors, National Top Think Tank Council, Chinese Academy of Social Sciences.

means of network will continue to be the main feature of post COVID-19 globalization. But the significance of globalization to world development remains unchanged because it is human nature to have communication and connection, which are the ways to fulfill happiness. This feature has never changed since the beginning of time. The only change is that the happiness index of human beings is higher and higher. Thus globalization will not stop after the pandemic but will be presented in a brand-new, enriched form and benefit people all over the world.

Globalization, as a sure way to pursue a happy life, has been widely recognized by people around the world. This is not only the vitality of globalization but also the source power of its future development. However, we must be aware that for quite a long time, the question of whether globalization has a future has aroused widespread concern in the international community. Among them, the American factor is the main cause of confusion. As the largest developed country in the world, the US has turned the clock back, changing its foreign policy from global expansion to isolationism. Hence the Establishment who stand for the former policy and the Conservative who support the latter are increasingly divided. The US is losing the willingness to lead as the cost of maintaining leadership in the international community is rising. Yet it is reluctant to allow other countries to be a supplement to its role. With the rise of new international forces, it has begun to reassess the efficiency of its open and multilateral international rules in safeguarding its interests, altering its policy from the "global model" to a semi-closed or even closed "club model". The view of world order and international norms led by American liberalism emphasizes the universality of American samples, without recognizing the geopolitical logic based on the strength of major countries, which, to some extent, leads to disputes and conflicts between the US and other major countries. As the mainstream Western values are questioned, Western societies are further divided, as exemplified by not only the split within the elite but also in the policy division between the Conservative and the Liberal Establishment, as well as the perception differences and contradictions between the elite and the public. Therefore, the worry about deglobalization prevalent in the international community for a period of time is indeed the uncertainty caused by the changeable US policy and multilateralism. This hallmark has been fully displayed by the current fight against COVID-19. A classic example is that at the press conference on May 29th, US President Trump turned a blind eye to more than 100000 deaths caused by the pandemic as well as the police's bloody killing of a black man; rather, he kept shifting the blame and insisted on decoupling. In this sense, the post-coronavirus globalization will no longer be solely dominated by America. Instead, there will be a win-win situation in which various players collaborate and consult with each other.

The obstructed US-led globalization and the rise of the conservative in the West will affect international order and norms in various fields. Despite many variables and uncertainties, China is faced with more opportunities than challenges on the whole. China's performance in the fight against COVID-19 is obvious to the international community. The "scores" of the battle against the coronavirus prove that the moral high ground and soft power of the US as a leader are no longer the same as what they once were. In terms of multilateral cooperation and global governance, the US is unwilling to take the lead in globalization and global governance, which provides an opportunity for China to take the moral high ground of global governance and free trade. The chaos in the world, including the frequent internal conflicts in the West and the intensified strides in America, requires a new rising power like China to restore the balance.

Recently, two pieces of news help to predict the trend in globalization. On May 27, German Chancellor Angela Merkel said in her public speech that the 27-member bloc's relationship with China would be a top priority of her government. "We Europeans will need to recognize the decisiveness with which China will claim a leading position in the existing structures of the international architecture", she said. Merkel reiterated her aim to complete an investment accord with China, as well as conducting close cooperation in fighting climate change and global health challenges. On May 30, Singapore's *Lianhe Zaobao* said an article that the 10 ASEAN countries and China promised to keep their markets open and refrain from imposing unnecessary trade restrictions. Previously on May 29, ASEAN and China issued the "Joint Statement on Combating the Coronavirus Disease (COVID-19) and Enhancing ACFTA Cooperation", reaffirming their commitment to work closely in the fight against this pandemic and calling for joint efforts in mitigating the impact of the pandemic on global and regional trade and investment. ASEAN and China commit to share anti-pandemic information and experience in a prompt and efficient manner, facilitate production and access to medicines and vaccines used for the treatment of COVID-19, and demonstrate the spirit enshrined in the ASEAN-China Strategic Partnership for Peace and Prosperity. On May 23, when visiting the economic members of the National Committee of the CPPCC during the "Two Sessions", President Xi Jinping re-emphasized, "We must promote technological innovation as well as other aspects of innovation, and advance the digital economy, smart manufacturing, life health, new materials, and other strategic emerging industries. We also need to create more new growth points and growth poles, manage to smooth all links of production, distribution, circulation, and consumption. In this way, we can gradually form a new development pattern in which the domestic circulation plays a leading role, with international circulation as a supplement and cultivate new advantages in international cooperation and competition under new circumstances." Merkel's statement on behalf of the EU and the joint statement of ASEAN-China economic ministers reflect the determination of the three major economies to jointly promote a new round of globalization and depict a diversified blueprint for future globalization. General Secretary Xi's important speeches at the "Two Sessions", which demonstrate China's steely determination to persevere in reform and opening up, reassure the world. The prospect of globalization featured by diversified development and win-win cooperation will hence be brighter and deliver more benefits to people of the world.

"一带一路"倡议：2.0版的全球化

胡北思（Marek Hrubec）*

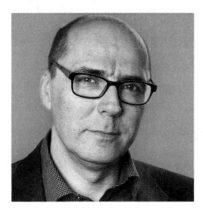

疫情大流行加速了历史。如其他类似的历史事件一样，它揭示并深化了已经存在的问题。因此，在疫情大流行期间，美中贸易摩擦或相关的全球互动都不会改善。但是，目前的情况既有问题，也有积极的方面。在当今世界发生深刻变化的时代，中国在未来一段时间内要比美国准备得更充分。

积极的方面是今天的疫情大流行与2008年金融和经济危机的情形存在区别。这次疫情在短期内几乎终止了许多国家的经济活动，这比2008年国际金融危机的影响更大。但是，现在并非经济原因导致经济放缓，而是源于非经济因素的病毒。因此，从长期看，只要病毒逐步消失，全球经济就可以反弹。许多国家已经开始恢复经济活力。

但形势不会再完全回到其最初状态。2500年前，欧洲哲学家赫拉克利特说过："人不能两次踏进同一条河流。"河流奔涌不息，时时不同。预计2020年许多国家的GDP将下降，下一年则有很大不确定性。

此外，由于此前时代以及疫情期间的经验，一些国家期望重塑全球化。他们发现，20世纪80年代美国和英国发起，仍然在一定程度

* 胡北思，捷克科学院全球化研究中心主任。

上起作用的最初版本的全球化，既带动了强大的全球经济联系，也引发了各种问题以及国际金融和经济危机。

现在，中国提供了具有创新性的2.0版全球化。这一全球化基于中国的"一带一路"倡议。该倡议自2013年提出以来，推动全球互动进入了新阶段。"一带一路"倡议做出了重要贡献，因为它在历史上源于中国文明独特的长期发展。自1978年以来，中国的改革开放一直在沿着"一带一路"、沿着历史悠久的丝绸之路前行。改革开放和以往的历史发展，是"一带一路"倡议的必要条件。因此，"一带一路"倡议是合乎中国发展逻辑的结果，它遵循了历史上形成的需求、利益、价值和可能性。

"一带一路"倡议致力于在世界参与伙伴相互承认基础上进行合作，为发展和多极化世界做出了重大贡献。"一带一路"倡议以亚欧大陆和东非为模板发展起来，然后拓展到世界其他地区。由于也涵盖拉丁美洲，因此这是一个全球性倡议，并因而在人类命运共同体概念中得以体现。

"一带一路"非常贴合新替代方案的全球趋势。我们最近目睹了单边主义的孤掌难鸣，同时也看到中国等国家在过去几十年中正在引入一种多极化观念。这不仅限于金砖国家，还包括墨西哥、印度尼西亚、土耳其，以及宏观区域性倡议，如上海合作组织、欧亚经济联盟、亚洲基础设施投资银行等。

特定的动因也将推动"一带一路"倡议在某个特定时刻落地：这与2008年后几乎在全球范围蔓延的经济和金融危机的后果在时间上交汇，尤其是美国等西方国家的危机，拖累了许多其他国家的经济与之一同下行。

自2008年危机爆发以来，西方国家对中国商品的需求一直呈下降趋势。由于中国经济是出口导向型的，中国政府在危机发生期间努力帮助中国公司，并扭转这一趋势。为了抵消国际经济危机的影响，中国政府投入资金推动和支持国内的公共基础设施以及其他项目建设，而在西方市场持续数年的不确定性之后，中国政府也开始活跃于国际和跨国领域。2013年宣布的"一带一路"倡议是创造性尝试，以一种与21世纪相适应的新形式重塑了历史悠久的丝绸之路。由于

"一带一路"倡议是在前一次危机之后提出的，因而为应对新型冠状病毒危机做好了充分准备。

尽管如此，美国总统仍然在以疫情大流行为借口，试图与中国进一步脱钩。他力图阻止各国与中国合作。有些国家可能会屈服。但大多数国家已经认识到哪种体系能、哪种体系却不能应对新型冠状病毒危机。就疫情控制而言，美国是世界上表现最糟糕的国家，这是其总体性衰落的一个表征。

相反，1978 年后的改革开放扎根并改造了中国。2014 年是美国 140 多年来（自 1872 年以来）首次失去对中国在世界 GDP（PPP）中所占份额的优势地位。现在，中国作为一个重要国家和文明类型已重返世界舞台。

发展中国家尤其注意到中国在过去 40 年间努力改善了基础设施，使 8 亿多人口摆脱了贫困。此外，中国还发展了高科技经济和社会。毫无疑问，世界上的发展中国家和发达国家都有与中国合作的动力。这是后疫情时代的一个良好起点。（于海青翻译）

原文：

"Chinamerica" Will be Replaced by the Belt and Road Initiative

Marek Hrubec[*]

The pandemic has accelerated history. Like other similar historical e-

———————
* Marek Hrubec, Director, Centre of Global Studies in the Institute of Philosophy at the Czech Academy of Sciences.

vents, it reveals and deepens the problems that already existed. Therefore, neither the US-China trade frictions nor related global interactions could be expected to improve during the pandemic. However, the current situation includes both problematic and positive aspects. In the contemporary era of profound world changes, China is much better prepared for the coming period of time than the USA.

The positive side is the difference between today's pandemic situation and the situation of the 2008 financial and economic crisis. On the one side, this time economic activities almost stopped in many countries in a short run as a consequence of the pandemic which was a bigger impact than in the 2008 global financial crisis. However, there is no economic reason of the economic slowdown now. It is a non-economic viral cause. Therefore, as soon as the viral cause disappears step by step, global economy can rebound almost fully in the long-term. It already started revitalizing in many countries.

However, things never return totally to their original state. The European philosopher Heraclitus said 2500 years ago: "No man ever steps in the same river twice." River flows; and it is not the same in a moment. A drop of GDP is expected in many countries this year, and next year is uncertain.

Moreover, due to the previous era and also due to the pandemic experience, some countries want to reshape globalization. They see that the first version of globalisation, which was initiated by the US and the UK in the 1980s and is still working to some degree, delivered not only strong global economic interconnections, but also triggered various problems and financial and economic crises around the world.

Now China offers something innovative: Globalisation 2.0. It is based on the China's Belt and Road Initiative (BRI) which has brought, above all, a new stage of global interactions since 2013 when it was established. The BRI has made a relevant contribution as, historically, it stems from the unique long-term development of China's civilization. China's reform and opening up since 1978 was already going down the path of the Belt and Road, following the historical Silk Road. The reform and opening up, in tandem with previous historical developments, were necessary conditions of BRI. Therefore, BRI has been a logical consequence consistent with Chinese developments, and follows historically shaped needs, interests, values, and possibilities.

The BRI has contributed significantly to the development and multipolar world by efforts to cooperate on the basis of mutual recognition of participating partners in the world. The BRI has been developed as a model in Eurasia and Eastern Africa, before going to other parts of the world. Since it has encompassed also Latin America, it is a global project. In this way, it is indicated in the concept of a community of shared future for mankind.

It fits well the global tendencies of new alternatives. While we have recently witnessed faltering unilateralism, at the same time we can see China and other countries introducing a multipolar perspective last decades. This is not limited to the BRICS countries but also includes Mexico, Indonesia, Turkey, for example, and also macro-regional initiatives, such as the Shanghai Organization of Cooperation, the Eurasian Economic Union, the Asian Infrastructure Investment Bank, etc.

There was also the specific motivation driving the establishment of the BRI at a particular moment in time, i. e. the time coincidence with the consequences of the economic and financial crisis playing out almost globally since 2008, particularly the crisis in the US and other Western countries, which dragged the economies of many other countries down with them.

Since the 2008 crisis erupted, Western countries' demand for Chinese goods has experienced a downtrend. As the Chinese economy was export-oriented, the Chinese government was keen to help Chinese companies at the time of crisis, and reverse the trend. Promoting and financially supporting public infrastructure and other projects in China as a counterbalance to the consequences of the global economic crisis, the Chinese government also started being active in the international and transnational spheres after several years of uncertainty on Western markets. The announcement of the Belt and Road Initiative in 2013 was a creative effort to reinvent the historical

Silk Road in a new form appropriate for the 21st century. Therefore, the Belt and Road Initiative is very well prepared to the coronavirus crisis because it was created after the situation of the previous crisis.

Nevertheless, the US president is using the pandemic as an excuse for greater decoupling with China. He seeks to discourage various countries from cooperating with China now. Some may actually bow. But most countries already see which system is capable of coping with the coronavirus crisis and which system is not. The United States is the worst country in the world when it comes to pandemic control. It is a symbol of its decline in general.

On the contrary, the reform and opening up since 1978 took root and transformed China. In 2014, this was the first time in more than 140 years (since 1872) that the USA had lost its primacy as for China's share of world GDP (PPP). Now China is back on the world stage as a major country and civilization.

Developing countries in particular see that China has managed to develop its infrastructure and lift more than 800 million people out of poverty over the last 40 years. In addition, China has developed its high-tech economy and society. There is no doubt that the motivation for cooperation with China exists for developing and developed countries around the world. This is a good starting point for the post-pandemic era.

国际秩序

疫情对国际政治体制前所未有的考验

托米斯拉夫·尼科利奇（Tomislav Nikolić）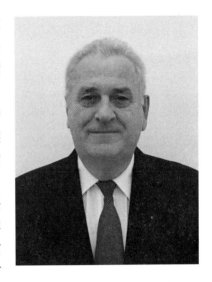*

　　毫无疑问，未来将会出现更多流行性疾病，不管是已知疾病及其危险的变体，还是全新的疾病，这些疾病必将势如破竹地席卷全球。

　　造成这一现状的根源是我们对待地球的粗暴方式。气候变化源于人类对完整植物群和野生动物食物链的破坏。

　　当我们为了获取肥沃的土地而去砍伐亚马孙雨林，为了耕种而征用非洲大草原，或去捕猎野生动物致使它们濒临灭绝时，我们以强取豪夺的方式接触到了以往从未接触过的真正大自然。我们征服了未知的领地，我们未曾在这些地方留下成长的痕迹，也从未面对面接触过它，当然也就完全不了解生存在这种环境中的微生物。因此，对这些微生物我们没有任何免疫能力。我们征服世界每一个角落的野心越大，感染上流行性疾病的可能性也越高。

　　此次新冠肺炎疫情是大自然对人类长期无视生态危机的一次回应，也可以说是一种防御机制，甚至是一次报复行为。

　　自第二次世界大战至今，大多数西方国家的人民从未经历过如此

---

　　* 托米斯拉夫·尼科利奇，塞尔维亚前总统、塞尔维亚对华对俄全国合作协调委员会主席。

严峻的威胁。这些疫情迫使他们对日常的生活、生产和消费做出翻天覆地的变化。我们曾一起目睹了多次自然灾害、大型集会抗议、若干国家体制机制的崩溃、个别国家恃强凌弱和若干次政治危机等，但事件发生后许多人的生活终究回归了正轨。

欧洲国家坐山观虎斗，见证了战争、干旱、政变、革命和传染病疫情，大多只是通过呼吁、捐赠、示威或军事手段间接参与。然而这一次，危机也迫在眉睫，改变了我们的生活方式。

随着新冠肺炎疫情肆虐整个世界，欧洲成为新的疫情中心。西方人的生活方式受到了当代史上前所未有的巨大影响。当然，这次疫情的破坏程度与世界大战无法相提并论。但是，在许多国家，人们的生活陷入了停滞。商店、咖啡厅、酒吧和餐馆都歇业了。机场和商场空无一人。几乎是一夜之间，生活方式发生了剧变。

现在看来，西方世界似乎无力改变固有的处理方式，并有效地应对此次疫情。新自由主义的教条忽视了自身的主要利益，资金流和企业利益把握着一切事物的命脉，国家无法施加任何影响。

对那些秉持着自由资本主义，并由软弱、混乱、毫无威信的政府领导的国家，这次新冠肺炎疫情像是一记警钟，号召人类选择其他发展道路。

以西班牙为例，新冠肺炎疫情在该国彻底暴发后，该国才正式通过了一项法案，允许国家接管全国范围内的私立诊所用于医疗救治。这种做法违背了自由贸易原教旨主义的基本原则和思想。这次疫情结束后，我们还能坚持这么做吗？全球范围的经济衰退正在发生。一方面，这次疫情可能演变成一连串的战争，造成独裁专制加剧，经济不公的现象越发明显；另一方面，疫情也可能促使我们抓紧行动，对危机应对体系进行转型优化。

我们为什么不能做些什么来应对气候变化？我们明明知道可以依据现有的生活方式转变、组织经济和社会体系，为什么还会执迷不悟，抱守现状，导致蒙受致命损失？

这次新冠肺炎疫情揭露了短视的个人主义社会体系的缺点。从全球范围来看，过去几十年针对感染病和疫情研究的投资项目有所减少，因为这些研究无法为医疗公司带来快钱，无法使公司股价飙升。

医疗公司宁愿将资金投向心脏病、焦虑症和性功能障碍等方面的研究。

美国副总统迈克·彭斯（Mike Pence）已被任命为美国应对新冠肺炎疫情工作组组长。但在他就任印第安纳州州长时，他曾主导大幅削减公共卫生基金，削减艾滋病毒检测能力，这一举措导致艾滋病在印第安纳州大量传播。同样地，2016年大选以后，特朗普政府削减了联邦政府对流行病防疫的资助。依据特朗普的一份声明，美国甚至将冻结一笔投向世界卫生组织的巨额资助。

在资本主义晚期，对公共医疗进行投资从商业角度看是不可持续的。考虑到医疗行业的准备情况以及医疗物资的库存情况，这次新型冠状病毒使全世界大开眼界。这次疫情表明，凡事顺其自然则万事大吉，一旦遇到危机则土崩瓦解。零售商处的呼吸机、防护口罩和抗菌产品迅速脱销，不久全国各地都买不到了，这种情况之前从未出现过。在平日里，没有人会投资库存或仓库以补充货架上的货物，即便有这样的需求也大多采购自中国以外的国家。而现在，许多国家需要订购相关产品，只得等待产品产出并交货。在这种不平等、不安全的情况下，保护大众的健康已变成不可能完成的任务。

新自由主义横行无阻多年以后，我们逐渐意识到，尤其在这次疫情面前，我们的安全、健康和繁荣更多有赖于一个强大的、设备精良的公共服务体系，而不是那些跨国公司。在医生、护士和其他医务工作者不辞辛劳、不遗余力地抢救生命的同时，跨国公司的亿万富豪们却躲在了豪宅的庇护所里。财富的再分配、税收公平和对社会层面的关注现在已经成为国家安全的重要议题。数据显示，此次疫情将导致全球贫困率上升，这是30年间的头一回。新冠病毒肺炎对国民经济的威胁比造成的公共卫生风险大得多。经济衰退可能使全球5亿人陷入贫困。截至4月10日，新型冠状病毒引发的死亡人数接近10万人，超过160万人确诊。疫情肆虐导致股市低迷、俄罗斯与沙特打起了石油价格战、叙利亚内战演变成潜在的移民危机，各种因素交织，致使数千万人丢了工作。如果不采取适当措施，新冠病毒肺炎可能在全球范围内引发持续数十年的经济崩溃。如果疫情不能得到控制，整个世界和现代秩序也可能消亡。

从目前的趋势来看，本次疫情以现代国际关系史上前所未见的方式对国际政治体制进行了考验。这场疫情最终可能为中国在国际舞台上赢得极高的道德权威。

新型冠状病毒、油价，甚至世界经济现状只是这场变革的注脚。这场变革与东西方间的权力平衡博弈有关。毫无疑问，美国已经主动放弃，或者说失去了全球领袖的位子。像许多西方自由主义民主国家一样，美国只关心如何处理好国内的新冠肺炎疫情。欧洲也正在采取与美国类似的做法。在应对新冠肺炎疫情的过程中，如果各国未能就采取共同的金融对策达成一致，那么欧盟未来的发展之路将变得凶险异常。西班牙、意大利和法国呼吁发行联合债券，将欧盟集团在市场上的借款集中起来，并为卫生部分和经济领域筹措额外的资金。但是德国和荷兰反对这一提议，两国解释称，这些举措将招致新的金融危机，欧元区及其成员国都会受到影响。有九个国家支持发行全欧范围内的通用债务工具，包括德国在内的四个国家则持反对意见。顺便说一句，这无关乎资源浪费，这是一个经济层面的生死存亡问题。欧盟各成员国尚未就危机应对方案达成共识。欧盟委员会主席乌苏拉·冯德莱恩（Ursula von der Leyen）想提出一个使欧盟各国生活正常化的路线图，但愤怒的欧盟各成员国首脑话都没听完便挂断了她的电话。

我们正面临着一个巨大的全球性问题。而最令人沮丧的是，欧洲和美国都没有展现出领袖该有的姿态。既然美国人当了逃兵，人们在想谁会站出来承担领袖的义务呢？至少有一件事情是肯定的，那就是纽约，即联合国不会站出来带头。

在习近平主席"一带一路"愿景的指导下，中国向所有受新冠肺炎疫情影响的国家捐赠了物资和设备，甚至派出了专家实地指导工作。这些举措在许多国家都受到了赞誉，这些国家也亲眼见证了中国治理模式的优越性。现在，人们明白了，如果一个国家教育好人民，并为不分贵贱的所有人提供医疗服务，那我们可以判定这个国家是富裕的。中国关心世界上所有受疫情影响的国家，同时深化与世界各国在安全、经济和政治领域的关系。从这些举动可以看出，中国正逐步展现真正的自我形象。

世界在变化。以前，每逢全球性的危机，美国总是第一个做出响应的国家，这为其赢得了声誉。现在，那些被贴上"霸权"标签的国家正主动为世界第一强国提供人道主义援助。有人认为，新冠肺炎疫情下的美国不再是那个我们之前所熟悉的美国了。这种观点恐怕要应验了。

塞尔维亚不站边。塞国对中华人民共和国所提供的援助表示无尽的感谢，尤其当疫情刚暴发，塞国内对该病毒知之甚少时，中国的医生来到塞尔维亚提供帮助。全世界所有国家都应该动议联合国大会通过一项决议，向中华人民共和国表示感谢，因为中国对武汉这座英雄的城市实施了全面的封锁，防止了疫情进一步蔓延。同时，多亏了中国领导人的英明决策，为全世界争取了一个月的宝贵时间，为抗击这场不可避免的灾难做好准备。（董方源翻译）

原文：

COVID-19：An Unprecedented Test of the International Political System

Tomislav Nikolić*

The future doubtlessly holds in store more epidemics of both the known diseases and their dangerous mutations, and of the completely new ones, which are bound to storm across the world without stopping.

The way we treat our planet is one of the main reasons behind this. The impact on climate change stems from the man's conduct towards the remaining intact flora and his fauna impoverishing treatment of the wild nature.

* Tomislav Nikolić, Former President, Serbia.

119

When we deforest the Amazon to gain fertile soil, claim the African savannah for the sake of farming, or hunt out wild animals to the brink of extinction, we interact uncompromisingly with the genuine wilderness that we have never been in touch with before. We conquer the swathes of nature that we do not know, as we have not grown up with it, or we have never been face-to-face with it, being of course completely ignorant of the microorganisms that live in such surroundings. Therefore, we are not immune to them. The more we strive to tame every corner of wilderness in the world, the more we fall victims to epidemics.

The COVID-19 pandemic is one of nature's responses to the long-ignored unfolding ecological crisis, if not a defence mechanism, or even revenge.

From WWII to this day, residents of most Western countries have not faced a threat serious enough to compel them to make a sea change in their lifestyle revolving around production and consumption. We witnessed a number of major protests, crumbling of states, a couple of attacks of the mighty against the weak, a handful of political crises and a few natural disasters, but life evolved normally for many.

The Europeans would observe the wars, droughts, coups, revolutions and epidemics from afar, only taking part indirectly, by means of appeals, donations, demonstrations, or militarily. Nowadays, however, the crisis is on our doorstep and is changing the way we live.

With the ravaging effects of the COVID-19 pandemic and Europe being the new hotspot, everyday Western life has been disturbed in the ways unprecedented in recent history. The destruction level is of course nowhere near the scale we saw in the world wars. Nevertheless, life has been reduced to a standstill in many countries. Shops, cafes, bars and restaurants are closed. Airports stand desolate. Business quarters are deserted. Lifestyle has changed almost overnight.

It seemed that the Western world was incapable of altering its ways and responding to threats efficiently. The neoliberal dogma is oblivious to the man and his interests, everything being in the hands of corporate interests and financial flows, devoid of any state impact.

The aftermath of the COVID-19 pandemic in the countries ruled by liberal capitalism, coupled with the weak, chaotic and unconvincing governments are a wake-up call for the mankind to take another route.

It took the outbreak of the COVID-19 pandemic for Spain to pass a law enabling the state to take over all private clinics country-wide for the purpose of medical treatment, this being in direct contravention of the basic principles and ideology of the free-trade fundamentalism. Are we capable of conducting ourselves like this once the current crisis is over? A global economic recession is underway. On the one hand, this could spiral into to a spate of wars, intensified dictatorship and a growing economic injustice, or it could empower us to call for the sorely needed transformation of the crisis-struck system.

Why cannot we do anything to combat climate change? Why would we revert to the fatal status quo when we know that we can transform and organize our economy and society according to the way we live right now?

The COVID-19 pandemic has unveiled the weaknesses of the short-sighted individualistic social system. Globally speaking, the past decades have seen a drop in investments aimed at the research of infectious diseases and pandemics, for this does not generate quick profits and a spike in the stock value to the companies operating in the health sector. They rather invest in the research of heart conditions, anxiety problems the treatment of impotence, etc.

In the capacity as Governor of Indiana, US Vice President Mike Pence, who has been appointed to head the COVID-19 response task force, initiated substantial cuts in the public health funds and HIV testing, which caused a massive spread of AIDS in the state.

Similarly, following the 2016 elections, Donald Trump's administration trimmed back the federal funds for the prevention of pandemics. Judging by a statement made by Mr. Trump, the US will even freeze a significant amount of funding to the World Health Organization.

Public healthcare investments are commercially unsustainable in late capitalism. This virus has been an eye-opener for the whole world vis-a-vis the preparedness of healthcare and the amount of stocks. It showed that everything is all right when things go their way, and that everything falls apart in times of crisis. Never has this been more obvious than in the case of ventilators, protective face masks and antibacterial products that quickly went out of stock at retailers, and then nationally. Against a lulling backdrop of the serene daily routine, no investments were made in stockpiles or warehouses to replenish the shelves from-it is necessary to order the products, wait for them to be made and delivered, often from no other country but China.

Protection of health as a public good has become impossible with this level of inequality and insecurity.

After years of unlimited neoliberalism, we have realized, in the face of this pandemic, that our security, well-being and prosperity hinge more heavily on the strong and well-equipped public services, than on multinational corporations. While doctors, nurses and other medical workers exert themselves tirelessly to save our lives, billionaires from multinational organizations have found asylum in their shelters. Redistribution of wealth, fair taxation and placing greater emphasis on the social aspect are now a matter of national security.

Data indicate that global poverty will rise for the first time in thirty years. The economic danger inherent in COVID-19 is exponentially higher than the risk to public health. Economic fallout of the COVID-19 epidemic might push half a billion people world-wide into poverty.

To this day, 10th April, 2020 the coronavirus death toll is nearly 100 thousand, with more than 1. 6 million confirmed cases, while dozens of millions will be economically deprived, especially due to the fact that the epidemic has created a perfect storm with the stock market downturns, the oil price war between Russia and Saudi Arabia, and the turning of the real war in Syria into a potentially emerging migrant crisis.

COVID-19 could cause a global economic collapse to last for generations if adequate measures are not taken; the world and the modern-day order could vanish if we fail to halt it.

Judging by the current trend, the pandemic has already put the international political system to the test in an unprecedented way in the modern history of international relations. The epidemic could end in Beijing gaining the supreme moral authority on the world stage.

This has to do with something much bigger than the coronavirus, the price of oil, or even global economy. This has to do with the balance of power between the East and the West.

The US has undoubtedly given up or lost the role of the global leader. Like many liberal democracies, it is solely concerned with the settlement of its own problems with COVID-19.

A process similar to the one in the US is playing out in Europe as well.

The future of the European Union will be put to danger if countries fail to agree on a joint financial response in the struggle against COVID-19.

Spain, Italy and France are calling for the issuance of joint bonds to pool the bloc's borrowing on the market and raise additional funds for the health sector and the economy, while Germany and the Netherlands oppose this, explaining that it could usher in a new financial crisis looming over the Eurozone and its respective economies.

Nine countries were in favour of the Europe-wide common debt instrument, while four, including Germany, were against it. By the way, this has nothing to do with obstinate wastefulness, but sheer economic survival.

EU Member States have so far been unable to agree on the way to overcome the crisis. EC President Ursula von der Leyen wanted to present a roadmap to normalizing life in the EU, but angry EU heads of state and government cut her short in a telephone conversation.

We have an enormous global problem at hand. What is most frustrating is that no gestures of leadership have come from either the European or the US side. Having in mind the absence of American leadership, everyone keeps wondering from where it will come. One thing is for certain—New York, i. e. the United Nations, will not take the lead.

The donations, equipment and experts sent by China to all the states hit by COVID-19, in the light of the Belt and Road vision promoted by President Xi Jinping, were met favourably in many countries that can witness the superiority of the Chinese governance model firsthand. Now one can see that a country is wealthy if it educates its people and provides them with medical care, be they rich or poor. China is showing its true self through its concern for all the affected in the world, while deepening its relationship with governments from across the globe in areas of security, economy and politics.

The world is changing. The US has always had a reputation of a first responder in every global crisis, and now the countries labelled authoritarian deliver humanitarian aid to the most powerful country in the world, at its own request. Those who think that the US as we know it will not be the same in the wake of COVID-19 are probably right.

Serbia does not participate in global divisions. It has expressed its boundless gratitude to the People's Republic of China for its assistance, especially for the fact that the Chinese doctors have come to Serbia to lend a helping hand in the struggle we knew little about. The way to go for all the countries in the world is to have the UN General Assembly approve a Resolution expressing gratitude to the People's Republic of China for placing the heroic city of Wuhan under a complete lockdown, owing to the wise decision of its leadership, thus affording us a month of preparation for the struggle against the scourge that was inevitable.

后疫情时代，世界将走向何方？

伊日·帕劳贝克（Jiří Paroubek）*

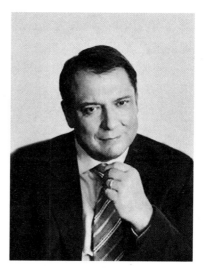

新冠肺炎疫情的迅猛来袭震惊了全世界，但这实质上是一场防御战。超载的地球正在抵御一场来自人类圈的攻击：人类滥用自己的新能力，试图从根本上改变地球的自然力量之比。我们必须尊重这一事实。同样基于这一事实，罗马俱乐部联合主席桑德琳·迪克森·德克塞夫说："新型冠状病毒对整个世界的影响表明，整个地球、所有物种、所有国家和地缘政治任务都是紧密相连的。除新型冠状病毒外，气候变化、生物多样性减少和金融危机也没有国家边界之分。当我们寻找其他星球的时候，就会意识到自己的所作所为。乱砍滥伐、生物多样性减少和气候变化都提高了疫情的风险。乱砍滥伐拉近了野生动物与人类的距离，增加了人畜共患病毒跨界传播的可能。为了发展自然导向型、公共福利型绿色循环经济，我们需要找到事情发生的诱因。"

在那些关注地球资源限制的人看来，上述问题似乎比当下威胁人类的健康问题更加宽泛，但太过宏观。例如，谈到公共福利型经济时，我立马注意到有必要扭转近几十年的趋势：几十个最富有的家庭

* 伊日·帕劳贝克，捷克共和国前总理。

拥有世界一半的财富。如果想要消除社会不平等，参与全球合作的各个经济体就不能采取"竞次"策略，即通过低工资、减税和短时监管来追逐利益。我们已经认识到，经济表现的衡量标准受到纯粹利益的误导，而它背后则是不计其数的破坏。

我们眼下还没有针对新型冠状病毒的药方，但对"竞次"的药方却有一定了解。G20 会议、达沃斯世界经济论坛及其他关注紧迫议题的场合，经常会讨论这些药方。不幸的是，这些讨论要么囿于学术层面，要么无法达成一致行动。单个公正的国家改变不了世界，尽管我并未低估榜样的力量。为了更持久的改变，至少需要一群强大的、愿意合作的国家，通过考量自身在世界经济中的经济份额，共同推动问题的解决。

正如布里埃尔·祖克曼或托马斯·皮凯蒂所建议的那样，唯有一个合作性的经济强国群体，才能使用更广泛统一的税基和共同金融财富登记来干预减税、逃税行为和避税港。这一群体将会发现税收陷阱在哪儿，谁在逃避纳税义务，以及在哪儿逃避。然后，它将采取共同的海关保护措施来打击避税港、防止不公平竞争。拒绝团结（其根源在于，贪婪是经济发展的主要动力）将把我们的星球变成地狱。

这些话看似与疫情无关，但也表明当前危机的解决不仅有赖于医学研究力量的壮大，也有赖于（各国）以负责任的态度遵从流行病学家和卫生学专家的建议。正如其他巨大灾害一样，这也是一个从根本上带来改变的良好契机，一个促使人们从更尖锐的角度看待环境压力的契机。即便是世界上最自由主义的政府也开始断然采取广泛社会措施，这是我们过去在左翼选举获胜以后也从未看到过的事情。人们意识到，倘若有人无法承担医疗检测费用、居家隔离或照顾突然停课的孩子，新型冠状病毒就将迎来新的暴发，并带来更猛烈的打击。

因此，团结和公平不仅是道德问题，也与人类的生存息息相关。当新型冠状病毒传递这一信息的时候，各国政府毅然抛却了对预算的过度忧虑，开始提供补贴或贷款担保，动用社会政策工具。其中，最广为人知的工具是短时工作，即政府支付部分工资，以防因需求剧减而导致私营公司裁员的情况发生。此举还有别的好处，它使我们想起进步左翼的梦想——全民基本收入。如果我们能够应用使人类远离机器的人工智能机器人，就将安然度过疫情。

但如果一些国家只能小范围使用上述团结工具，可能也会导致不公平。这正是欧盟特别是南欧国家倡议使用欧盟共同基金（而不光是国家财政）为这些政策提供融资的原因。自 2008/2009 年国际金融危机爆发以来，南欧国家始终没有摆脱政府债务的阴影。

一些领域的共同程序已然发生。欧盟委员会和欧洲议会已经支持欧洲央行与银行业合作，在风险时期向中小企业提供更灵活的贷款。根据欧盟委员会 2005 年 6 月 29 日发布的银行业计划，应加快经济自主工具（如"员工项目"）的使用。如果一家公司受到停业或投机性销售的威胁，则其员工可以把它变成受雇者或合作社所有权公司，这对员工无疑是一个新的机会。

世界各地采用的其他工具让我们想起 20 世纪 30 年代大萧条时期的"自下而上式"实践。正如贝尔纳德·列特尔所述，在大范围失业时期，出现了由地方生产负担的地方货币。奥地利煤城沃格尔在这方面起了先锋作用，其货币由煤矿来承担运营。这些货币的特点是：只能在当地使用，对当地生产进行估价，并使用"滞留费"，即时效价值，这有点像负利率。对于没有花掉的钱，人们通常会购买代币券，以便下个月使用。

中国地方政府（如武汉）发放的代币券也属于类似性质。它们可以用作地方购物，并具有时间限制，以鼓励钱的更快流通。这些工具的使用对地方经济生态是一个有益的补充，有助于人们抗过疫情。

地方化是关闭国家边界和保持社交距离的必然结果。疫情还推动了数字化的引入和机器人对人类的取代过程。印孚瑟斯总裁、世界经济论坛委员会委员莫希特·乔希留意到很多这样的变化。他说："灵敏度、扩展性和自动化是新商业时代的关键词，拥有这些能力的人将是当今的赢家。"

此次疫情凸显出数字化和远程合作的优势，使我们重新评估和塑造消费、供应、互动和生产的模式。数字化和远程合作不是崭新的事物，但却大大拓展了生产模式的分布式数字合作形式。根据工业 4.0 原则，数字化和远程合作可以在远程全球生产中心中得到应用。

通过引入全民基本收入要素，政府干预无意中加快了这一趋势，

127

从而使人类在福利未经削减的情况下被逐渐取代。这些中心规模很小，且能够服务于地方化需求。同时，小型地方经济体更适合当地人的承受能力，因而对经济自主化持开放态度。

生产和地理日趋多元化是构成（商业）韧性即抵抗力的要素。乔西强调指出，从长远来看，商业应当致力于提高韧性和反应时间。提高韧性的需要将迫使我们在供应链中逐步推广机器自动化和人工智能，以便减少接触，消除感染风险，降低对人工的依赖。生产和地理多元化还有助于及时对需求变化做出反应，以便增加或减少生产。

韧性、灵活度和处理突发变化的能力是所有战略的核心。乔西总结道，企业要看自己在哪些方面可以做得更强，哪些方面可以更加灵活。

后疫情时代的全球经济将会是什么样子？事实上，我们正在目睹一场针对不确定性所作的反应。早在 2008/2009 年国际金融危机期间，这种不确定性就已经在超全球化背景下出现，且程度越来越高。来自慕尼黑大学（凯末尔·基里克）和慕尼黑工业大学及经济政策研究中心（达莉亚·马林）的两位德国学者注意到了这一点。他们指出，早期的全球化实践（自 20 世纪 50 年代开始，将生产转向低成本国家）在"铁幕"消失和中国入世后，经历了大规模的扩张。交通革命即集装箱的广泛使用进一步推动了全球化进程。随着全球价值链的形成，我们开始步入超全球化阶段，该阶段仅在 2008 年国际金融危机期间中止过。在巅峰时期，全球价值链一度占到世界贸易增长的 60%。

经济学人智库报告指出，用机器人和人工智能来取代人类的强大动力并不是新近才出现的。报告认为，2011 年后，全球价值链的增长就已停滞，原因之一就是世界贸易不确定性的增加。在 2008/2009 年国际金融危机和 2012 年欧债危机期间，世界不确定性指数升高了 200%。根据该报告，世界不确定性指数主要是指不确定性或变化的表现频率。

2003 年"非典"暴发期间，世界不确定性指数增长了 70%。如果将世界不确定性指数与全球价值链数据联系起来，可以看出不确定性对富裕国家全球价值链的巨大影响。报告预计，新冠肺炎疫情可能导致不确定性增加300%，相应地，全球价值链活动也将减少35.5%。

世界经济的一个根本变化是制造业向富裕国家的回归。取代离岸的是其相反过程——回岸。新技术成本的下降正在彰显廉价工作的重要性。这将增加生产在附加值中的份额，但本身并不意味着对工人有利。报告认为，特朗普和新型冠状病毒都加快了世界劳动分工的变化，但真正的诱因却是2008/2009年的国际金融危机。

2014年，韩国和日本是机器人行业的领导者，每1000名工人中约有6个机器人，德国有4个，捷克、斯洛伐克和斯洛文尼亚有2个，美国有1.5个。那是中国强势崛起以前的事了。机器人和人工智能的到来并不意味着世界的分裂（除非下一届美国政府专注于此），但短距离物质生产将会是一个优先选择。该政策对发展中国家形成的重大冲击，需要各国协同应对。我们已经认识到需求，但还需要相互协调。（王文娥翻译）

原文：

Where the World Will Head After the Pandemic

Jiří Paroubek[*]

A new wave of risk has returned us to the need for sustainability and resilience care. There will also be an effort to shorten the ways of material production. The hard impact of this policy on developing countries requires a co-

* Jiří Paroubek, Former Prime Minister, The Czech Republic.

ordinated global response. We already know about the need, but we are yet to agree on a way.

The COVID-19 pandemic surprised the world with the speed and power of its attack, but it was actually a defense. The overloaded planet is defending against the aggressiveness of the anthroposphere, overusing humanity's new ability to fundamentally change the ratios of natural forces on Earth. The answer must come from respecting this fact. In this spirit also Sandrine Dixson-Declève, Co-President, The Club of Rome, said, "When we see how a single COVID-19 virus has affected the whole world, it is a demonstration of how the entire planet, all species, all countries or geopolitical tasks are interconnected. Not only coronavirus, climate change, biodiversity loss or financial collapse do not respect national borders. We have wake up to realize what we are doing when we go beyond planetary possibilities. Deforestation, biodiversity loss and climate change have increased the risk of the pandemic. Deforestation pushes wild animals closer to humans and increases the likelihood that zoonotic viruses like COVID-19 will cross the boundaries between species. We need to look for the causes of what happened and use it to implement green circular economy that is embedded in nature-based solutions geared towards the public good. "

The list of problems from the perspective of those who focus on the limits of planetary resources is at first glance much wider than the focus on the very health aspect of the current threat, but it is too general. For example, mentioning the need for an economy geared towards the public good, I immediately see the need to reverse the trend of recent decades, when several dozen wealthiest families have owned half the wealth of the planet. But if we want to eliminate unsustainable social inequalities, it is not possible for the main strategies of economies involved in global cooperation to be "races to the bottom," the search for benefits in low wages, tax undercutting and the most perishable regulation. We are beginning to feel how misguided the assessment of economic performance is by a single "bottom line" number, mere profit, while behind it results in uncounted damages.

While we do not have a drug against COVID-19 yet, anti race to the bottom drugs have been known for some time. They are often discussed, for example, at G20 meetings or at the World Economic Forum in Davos and on similar occasions when attention is focused on urging topics. Unfortunately, often only academically or without the ability to achieve coordinated action. One fair country will not change the world, though I do not underestimate the power of example. However, for a more lasting change, at least a group of strong cooperating countries is needed, which can push the agreed solution by weighing its economic share of the world economy.

Only a cooperative group of economically powerful states can intervene, for example, against tax undercutting, tax evasion and tax paradises by using a more broadly unified tax base and common financial wealth registers, as recommended by Gabriel Zucman or Thomas Piketty. They would find out where the tax traps are and who is running away from tax liability and where. They could then turn against unfair competition with common customs protection against tax paradises. With the term "paradise", be careful, after all. The refusal of solidarity to address common problems, the source of which is greed as the main engine of the economic movement, contributes to the fact that our planet has begun to turn into hell.

Those remarks, which seemingly fell out of the pandemic framework, illustrate that the current crisis is not only solvable by concentrating forces on medical research and by responsible compliance with the rules offered by epidemiologists and hygienists. Like any major shock, it is also an excellent opportunity for a fundamental change, to awaken to new conditions that allow the pressure of circumstances to be seen in a much sharper perspective. Even the most liberal governments around the world have suddenly begun to apply a whole range of social measures that we might not have seen even after the left's election victory. They realized that if a part of society could not afford to undergo a medical examination, stay at home in quarantine or with children who had suddenly closed school, coronavirus would take on new outbreaks and strike even more intensely.

Solidarity and justice, which are transformed into sufficient social care and justice, are therefore not only moral issues, but are among the limits whose disruption threatens the existence of the mankind. When the coronavirus explained this to governments again, they suddenly threw away excessive budgetary concerns, dictated by the surviving austerity policy, and reached for subsidies or loan guarantees, but also social instruments. The most popular is Kurzarbeit, where they pay a portion of wages to prevent the dismissal of employees from private companies due to the sharp decline in demand. There are also benefits reminding of the dreams of the progressive left, i. e. universal basic income. It can easily survive a pandemic if it establishes artificial intelligence robotics with no less ability to push people away from machines.

But even solidarity instruments can be a source of injustice if some countries can only use them on a lower scale. That is why initiatives are emerging in the EU, particularly in its southern wing, to finance these policies from the Common European Fund. That is, not just from state budgets, which in the south still suffer from debt from the days of the 2008/2009 global crisis.

Somewhere, the common procedure has already taken place. The European Commission and the European Parliament have supported the European Central Bank in coordinating the banking sector in promoting greater flexibility in lending, particularly for SMEs in times of increased risk. The European Commission's banking package of 29 June 2005 also includes a reference to the need to accelerate economic democracy instruments, such as "employee projects". This is a newly introduced opportunity to offer the company that is threatened with closure or speculative sales to employees and thus it can become an employee or cooperative ownership.

News from the world show that other instruments remind of the "bottom-up" practice dating back to the Great Depression of the 1930s. As Bernard Lietaer describes it, at the time of the huge unemployment, local currencies covered by local production were created. I know the pioneering example of the Austrian mining town of Woergel, where they were covered with mined coal. For these currencies and their followers, it was characteristic that they could been used only locally, they priced local production and used "demurrage", time limit values, something like negative interest. It was usually an obligation to buy a voucher for unspent money to use it another month.

And similar in nature are the current Chinese vouchers, which are now offered by local governments, for example in Wuhan. They include the advantage of local purchases as well as a time limit to encourage faster circulation of money. The introduction of these tools can also survive a pandemic because it is a suitable complement to the ecosystem of local economies.

Localization is one of the trends that inevitably emerges from the environment of the closure of state borders and social distancing. The epidemic has also accelerated the introduction of digitalisation and the replacement of humans by robots. Many of these changes were captured by Mohit Joshi, executive from Infosys Ltd., a member of the Council of the World Economic Forum. He says, "Agility, scalability and automation will be the watchwords for this new era of business, and those that have these capabilities now will be the winners."

The pandemic has highlighted the benefits of digitalisation and remote collaboration, which will force us to re-assessing and re-imagining modes of consumption, supply, interaction, and productivity. Let us add that this is not a complete novelty, but it is giving rise to a greater expansion, especially in the form of distributed digital cooperation on production templates, which can then be implemented in remote universal production centres according to the principles of Industry 4.0.

As the author points out, government interventions unintentionally accelerate this trend by introducing elements of universal basic income, allowing people to be gradually replaced without compromising their welfare. To this end, these centres can also be small and can serve localization needs. At the same time, smaller local economies are more affordable to the finances of the people who live there, so they are open to democratizing the economy.

Greater production and geographical diversification are elements of resilience, resistance, but not in combination with careful waiting. Joshi stresses that in the long term, businesses need to focus their attention on increasing resilience combined with response speed. The need to increase resilience will force us to increasingly implement the robotic automation and artificial intelligence in supply chains, which reduce the need to touch things, eliminate the risk of contagion, while reducing dependence on human presence. They also facilitate the response to a sudden change in demand when production needs to be increased or reduced.

Resilience finds itself at the forefront of any strategy, but also the agility and the ability to cope with unexpected change. Businesses need to look where they might be stronger and where they can be more flexible, Joshi sums up.

So, what will the global economy look like after the pandemic? In fact, we are witnessing an ongoing response to the growing uncertainty that emerged in the context of hyperglobalisation already during the 2008/2009 global crisis. This is highlighted by a pair of German researchers Kemal Kilic, LMU Munich, and Dalia Marin, Technical University of Munich; CEPR Research Fellow. They both work together in the European Digital Research Network, an internet-based tool for coordinating research at scattered European universities and research centres. As they point out, the earlier practice of globalization, which has shifted production to cheap countries since the 1950s, expanded substantially after the fall of the Iron Curtain and China's entry into the WTO. It also resulted from the transport revolution, i. e. the widespread use of containers. Global Value Chains (GVC) were created that took us to the hyperglobalisation phase, disrupted only by the 2008 financial crisis. In the peak period, GVC accounted for to 60% of world trade growth.

The Economist Intelligence Unit—EIU. Thus, strong incentives to replace humans with robots and artificial intelligence have arisen before. According to the authors, after 2011, GVC growth has already stopped. One reason was the increase in uncertainty in world trade. Between the 2008/2009 Global Crisis and the Euro Area Debt Crises 2012, the World Uncertainty Index increased by 200 percent. WUI is based on the frequency of expressions of uncertainty or variations in The EIU reports.

When SARS broke out in 2003, WUI grew by 70 percent. Linking WUI to GVC data then shows the huge impact of uncertainty on GVC in rich countries. As WUI grows, the share of imports from low-wage countriesin total inputs has fallen sharply. According to estimates by the authors of the paper, the COVID-19 pandemic is likely to increase the level of uncertainty by 300 percent according to WUI, reducing GVC activity by 35.5 percent.

A fundamental change in the world economy is the return of manufacturing to rich countries. Off-shoring is replaced by the opposite process, re-shoring. The fall in the price of new technologies is pushing the importance of cheap work. This will increase the share of production in added value, but that in itself does not mean that it is in favour of workers. Both Donald Trump and COVID-19 accelerated these changes in the world's labour division, but the real trigger was the Global Crises of 2008/2009, the authors note.

In 2014, South Korea and Japan were the leaders of robotics, with about 6 robots per 1000 workers, Germany 4, Czech, Slovakia and Slovenia 2, the United States 1.5. That was before China's decisive rise. The advent of robots and artificial intelligence does not mean that the world will begin to fall apart (unless the next US administrations are focused on this), but shorter distances in material production will be a priority where possible. The hard impact of this policy on developing countries requires a coordinated global response. We already know about the need, but we are yet to agree on a way.

对联合国系统的重新思考

何塞·路易斯·森特利亚·戈麦斯
（Jose Luis Centella Gomez）*

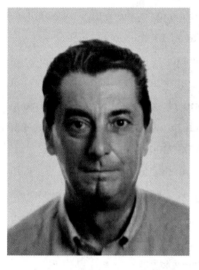

从《联合国宪章》中可以看出，设立联合国的最初意图是用其替代单边统治或权力均势的世界体系，从而得到一个以进步、自由和追求幸福为目标，以捍卫人权为纽带的集体安全体系。

为了明确这种集体安全体系，我们有必要先确定一下可能对人权保护造成威胁的事项，包括：

·经济问题和社会问题，尤其是贫困、传染病和环境恶化；

·气候变化；

·洲际冲突；

·内部冲突，包括内战、种族灭绝；

·核武器、放射性武器、生化武器；

·恐怖主义和有组织的国际犯罪。

《联合国宪章》的最初目标很快就被搁置了，并且被一种集团模式所取代。虽然谈不上阻碍，但它也为联合国工作的有效执行增加了难度。在实践中，联合国的组成和运作无论从结构上还是概念上都是

---

* 何塞·路易斯·森特利亚·戈麦斯，西班牙共产党主席。

按照这种集团模式发展起来的。

联合国的主要结构性问题体现在它只赋予了联合国大会几乎象征性的作用以及安全理事会的组成和权限，这从支撑"冷战"的均势体系和集团体系可见一斑。当然还包括联合国不同机构和计划之间缺乏协调，尤其是在与司法相关的机构之间，还有运作资源的缺乏。

联合国大会没有能力执行其决议，这些决议被交由安全理事会来处理。安全理事会可以发布具有约束力的决议，并动用国家军队来执行它们。这样，联合国安全理事会就变成了掌握实际权力的机构，其组成和运作规则仍然体现在冷战期间的世界体系中，还体现在五大常任理事会的否决权上。到 2009 年，安全理事会共遭到了 261 次否决，其中有 123 次来自苏联—俄罗斯，美国 82 次，英国 32 次，法国 18 次，中国 6 次。俄罗斯的否决权大多行使于 1950—1960 年，主要与国家准入相关。美国的否决主要与以色列和中东问题相关。

按照这种结构模式，联合国不可能确定和执行横向的国际治理模式，因为这意味着要接受新型多极国际秩序模式。因此，必须按照新的结构和运作规则来构建一种全新的国际组织模式。

很难想象，在当今世界上占有权力并享受为其量身定做的联合国系统的那些人会去推动他们自我转型。因此，有一种积聚力量为必要的改变打开通路的可能性，就是推动一场伟大的全球运动，为全人类的共同命运构建一种全球治理方案。

与同意需要建立"国际新秩序"的国家一道开展一场运动，民间社会可以通过各种集体和人民运动参与其中，并通过多元化媒体进行公开，以保障其透明度。

目标是提出一项在国家主权与国际合作之间取得平衡的提案，明确定义以尊重国家权力为出发点来处理国际问题的国际机构之间的权限，这些国家权力都是因承认国家主权而获得的。

根据对联合国作用的上述定义，修改联合国大会的组成、权限和运作方式使其决议不再是建设性的而是法律性的，同时改变经费的融资方式，可以根据每个国家的 GDP 来计算，这具有十分重要的意义。

要加强联合国大会的作用，必须同时降低安全理事会的权限，还要改变其组成方式，重新定义联合国的其他组织（国际法院、秘书处、托管理事会和经济及社会理事会）以及构成组织机构图的各个机构。

关于安全理事会，取消永久性成员的资格和是否可以对任何协议行使否决权，这两点至关重要，也就是构建一个其选举和权限都取决于联合国大会的新安全理事会，同时秘书处的地位与联合国的执行任务也应有更大的关联。

关于其他重要机构，应考虑是否能将国际法院和国际刑事法院统一在一个"国际法院"中，该法院以尊重各国主权为出发点，既包括一个负责国家间调解的法院，又包括一个专门审理国际罪犯的法院。

为了保障集体安全并应对前文所述的与经济发展不平衡、贫困等相关的威胁，需解决的基本问题在于结束世界银行和国际货币基金组织的工具化。它们目前不受联合国的任何控制，通过采用超自由政策和新殖民政策，它们已经变成了保证资本主义强国统治的工具。

必须采用具有平等和团结性质的新型经济和社会工具，以互惠互利为原则，在一个切实致力于推动全球特别是受惠较少的国家和地区社会经济发展的经济及社会理事会的框架下行动，这是一个民间社会广泛参与的与联合国大会关系最为紧密的经济及社会理事会，它在定义和发展新型国际经济体系时将发挥举足轻重的作用。目前，市场不但主导了经济，还主导了政治和社会生活，而这种新型国际经济体系将结束这种现状，让联合国大会和经济及社会理事会为市场运作设定整体路线，让经济政策惠及普遍利益。

其目标是让新型国际经济秩序服务于改善社会、教育、文化和卫生体系，从而进一步提高全人类的生活质量。

总之，在至少完成以下几个任务的基础上，通过为全球居民带来共同利益的多边世界治理模式来构建一个国际共同体，也就是构建一个全人类的共同项目：

- 为实现 2030 年的可持续发展目标而提出经济和社会发展计划；
- 捍卫每个人的所有人权；
- 摒弃父权社会，提高女性的地位；
- 在伦理观和道德观的基础上推动教育计划；
- 推动保障医疗卫生安全的计划。

在制定新型联合国模式时，有必要明确以横向性和多边性为特点的全球治理概念，即协调不同的政治和社会主体。因为人类的问题不能仅仅通过最高权力机构来解决，而是需要不同的参与者、政府和民间组织来开展明确和协调的行动，这一点已经越来越显而易见了。因此，集体安全必须从全球风险治理的角度来看待。为此，应当在不同的地区、国家、区域层次上开放空间，让与集体安全有关的各方都能参与讨论。

确定框架和参与性的难题在于将主角的位置还给联合国，因为其目前扮演的角色是受限制且无效的。除此之外还有一个难题，就是军事集团和国家集团拒绝放弃其在国际舞台中的主导地位而为多极世界让路。因此，应提议让联合国在建立更好和更安全的全球社会中发挥重要作用，以构建一些公正、有代表性和合法的国际机构，为全人类营造有利的社会和经济条件。

所以，还应提高那些依赖世界卫生组织、联合国儿童基金会、联合国开发计划署、世界劳工组织、联合国教科文组织的计划的有效性和重要性，这些计划如今正在遭受那些不接受多极世界关系模式的人的质疑和攻击。

总之，摒弃因冷战和地理因素而产生的受大国势力影响的模式，重新思考和修改联合国系统，这是一个至关重要的问题，不仅是为了有效应对全球威胁、风险和问题，也是为了赋予联合国至今未有的合法性。因此，我们要指出的一个基本问题是将联合国大会定义为一个凌驾于安全理事会和秘书处之上的国际立法机关，它应拥有行政权并赋予国际法院以权力。至于联合国是否应该拥有国际性质的武装部队，直接效力于联合国并受联合国大会的控制，这个争论还悬而未决。另一个基本问题是定义一系列附属机构，以执行经大会批准的各种计划，这些计划最终由国际货币基金组织和世界银行的大量资本来进行实际拟定、运作和控制。

最后重申，这种对联合国系统重新设计的模式不能从小处着眼，比如不同的国家主权，抑或是居民按照国际法规自由决定其经济、社会和文化体系的权利；相反，应该具备协调行动的职能，按照和谐的国际秩序和超越任何殖民主义残余的互惠互利基础上的关系来开展工作。

从这些角度来看，那些想在建设新世界和朝着野蛮毁灭地球之路继续前进之间做出抉择的人们，应该从对地球和大多数人有利的角度出发，意识到这个过程必须将政治提议、学术辩论与通过大规模调动群众来影响国际局势的能力结合起来。因为如果没有人民有组织的压力，就不可能达成国际共识，对联合国进行真正深刻的变革，为新型国际秩序开辟道路。毕竟我们很难相信，自苏联解体后，由北大西洋轴心主导的国际秩序会在不发动战争的情况下就接受其衰落。

在此范畴下，国际压力应该落在民间社会身上，由民间社会呼吁结束联合国的现状，因为联合国秘书长本人都承认，联合国没有对其必须应对的全球遭遇的多重人道主义危机、战争冲突和医疗卫生突发事件做出反应。因此，联合国的转型在很大程度上取决于人类在和平和可持续发展中前进的未来。（徐璞玉翻译）

原文：

Ideas Para Repensar el Sistema de NN. UU.

Jose Luis Centella Gomez *

La idea original de NN. UU. que plasmaron en su Carta Fundacional era reemplazar un sistema de dominio unilateral o de equilibrio de potencias, para conseguir un sistema de seguridad colectiva desde ideas de progreso, libertad y búsqueda de la felicidad con una vinculación referencial a la defensa de los Derechos Humanos.

Para concretar este sistema de seguridad colectiva habia que determinar las posibles amenazas de las que proteger a la humanidad, quedando

* Jose Luis Centella Gomez, President, Communist Party of Spain.

señaladas：

· Problemas económicos y sociales, destacando la pobreza, las enfermedades contagiosas y la degradación medioambiental.

· Cambio climático.

· Conflictos interestatales.

· Conflictos internos, incluyendo guerras civiles, genocidios.

· Armas nucleares, radiológicas, químicas y biológicas.

· Terrorismo y crimen internacional organizado.

Rápidamente los objetivos originales, la propia Carta Fundacional, fueron apartados y sustituidos por un esquema de bloques que dificultaba, cuando no impedía, efectuar sus tareas con eficacia, este esquema de bloques sobre el que se desarrollaron en la práctica tanto la composición como el funcionamiento de las NN. UU. contiene problemas tantos estructurales como conceptuales.

El principal problema estructural de NN. UU. es el papel casi simbólicoque se concede a la Asamblea General y la configuración y competencias del Consejo de seguridad con reflejo del sistema de equilibrios y bloques sobre el que se sustento la Guerra Fría, pero también incluye la descoordinación entre los diferentes organismos y programas de las NN. UU. , especialmente entre las instituciones relacionadas con la justicia, sin olvidar la escasez de recursos para el funcionamiento.

La Asamblea General no tiene capacidad para ejecutar sus resoluciones que se dejan en manos del Consejo de Seguridad que si pueden emitir resoluciones vinculantes y recurre a los ejércitos nacionales para su ejecución. De esta manera, el Consejo de Seguridad de NN. UU. se convierte en el organismo que tiene el poder real, con una composición y unas reglas de funcionamiento que siguen siendo un reflejo del sistema mundo vigente durante la guerra fría, reflejado en el derecho a veto de los cinco miembros permanentes, de esta manera, hasta 2009, el Consejo de Seguridad había sufrido el veto en 261 ocasiones 123 de la URRS-Rusia, 82 EE. UU. , 32 Reino Unido, 18 Francia y 6 china, la mayoría de los vetos rusos fueron ejercidos entre 1950 y 1960 relacionados con admisiones de países, mientras que los EE. UU. estan referidos a cuestiones relacionadas con Israel o el Oriente Medio.

Con este esquema estructural es imposible conseguir que las NN. UU. definan y ejecuten un esquema de gobernanza internacional de carácter horizontal, porque supondría aceptar un nuevo modelo de orden internacional multipolar siendo por lo tanto necesario construir un nuevo esquema de organización internacional, con nuevas estructuras y normas de funcionamiento.

No es fácil considerar que quienes en estos momentos detentan el Poder en el mundo y estan cómodos con un sistema de NNUU a su medida vayan a impulsar su propia transformacion, por ello la una posibilidad de acumular fuerzas para que se abran paso los cambios necesarios es impulsar una gran movimiento mundial sobre la necesidad construir una gobernanza global del Planeta para un destina común para toda la humanidad.

Un movimiento en la que junto a los Estados que estén de acuerdo en la necesidad de un Nuevo Orden Internacional puedan participar la sociedad civil, a través de todo tipo de colectivos y movimientos de carácter popular, así como la trasparencia garantizada por su apertura a los medios de comunicación de carácter plural.

El objetivo es plantear una propuesta que consiga una tensión equilibrada entre soberanía nacional y la cooperación internacional, defiendo claramente competencias entre instituciones internacionales que actuarían en cuestiones de incumbencia internacional desde el respeto a las competencias de cada Estado derivado del reconocimiento de la soberanía nacional.

En esta definición del papel de NN. UU. cobra toda su importancia una modificación de la composición, competencias y funcionamiento de la Asamblea General para que sus resoluciones dejen de tener carácter de recomendaciones y pasen a tener carácter de Ley, cambiando también las formas de financiación que podrían calcularse en función del PIB de cada Estado.

Potenciar el papel de la Asamblea General tiene que llevar emparejado la disminución de las competencias del Consejo de Seguridad, así como un cambio en su composición, y una redefinición del resto de organismos de NN. UU. (Corte Internacional de Justicia, secretaria, consejo de administración Fiduciaria y Concejo Económico y Social) así como de las distintas Agencias que completarian el organigrama.

Respecto al Consejo de Seguridad resulta imprescindible la desaparición de la condición de miembro permanente y la posibilidad de ejercer cualquier derecho de veto ante cualquier acuerdo, es decir un nuevo Consejo de Seguridad que sea dependiente en su elección y en sus competencias de la Asamblea General y que estaría acompañado de una mayor vinculación de la figura de la Secretaria General a las tareas ejecutivas de NN. UU.

En referencia a otros elementos importantes señalar la posibilidad de unificar la Corte Internacional de Justicia y la Corte Penal Internacional dentro de un Tribunal Internacional que contendría, por un lado, una corte encargada de mediar entre Estados y por toro una corte enfocada a juzgar a individuos que cometieran delitos de carácter internacional, desde el respecto a las distintas soberanías nacionales.

Cuestión básica para afrontar una de las amenazas señaladas como peligros para garantizar la Seguridad Colectiva, las relacionadas con los desequilibrios económicos, la pobreza etc. , es acabar con la instrumentalizacion del Banco Mundial y del Fondo Monetario Internacional, que sin control alguno desde NN. UU. , se han convertido en instrumentos para asegurar el dominio de las grandes potencias capitalistas mediante la aplicación de políticas ultraliberales y neocoloniales.

Son necesarios nuevos instrumentos económicos y sociales de carácter igualitario y solidario que actúen desde el principio del beneficio mutuo en el marco de un Concejos económico y social dedicado realmente a promover el desarrollo social y económico de todos los pueblos del Planeta, en especial de los Estados y territorios menos favorecidos, un consejo Económico y social dedicado realmente a promover el desarrollo social y económico de todos los pueblos del Planeta, en especial de los Estados y territorios menos favorecidos, un Consejo Económico y Social con participación de la sociedad civil mas relacionado con la asamblea General que tuviera peso a la hora de definir y desarrollar un nuevosistema económico internacional, que termine con la realidad actual de que el mercado domina no solo la economía, sino también la política y la vida, para que sea la Asamblea General de NN. UU. el Consejo Económico social quienes marquen las líneas generales al funcionamiento del mercado para conseguir que las políticas económicas sirvan al interés general.

El objetivo es poner el nuevo orden económico internacional al servicio de mejorar los sistemas sociales, educativos, culturales, sanitarios para conseguir mejorar la calidad de vida de toda la humanidad.

En definitiva, construir una Comunidad Internacional que pueda construir un proyecto comun para toda la humanidad, mediante un modelo de gobernanza mundial multilateral con benéficos compartidos para todos los pueblos del plantea, basado en conseguir al menos cuatro tareas:

· Proponer el desarrollo económico y social para cumplir los objetivos de desarrollo sostenible 2030.

· Defender todos los derechos humanos para todos los seres humanos.

· Mejorar la condición de la mujer enterrando la sociedad patriarcal.

· Promoción de programas educativos basados en valores éticos y morales.

· Promoción de programas que garanticen la seguridad médico-sanitaria.

En este desarrollo de un nuevo esquema de NN. UU. es necesario concretar la noción de gobernanza global de carácter horizontal y multilateral, que coordine a los diferentes agentes políticos y sociales porque cada vez es más evidente que los problemas de la humanidad no se pueden llevar exclusivamente a través de una autoridad suprema, sino que necesita una acción expresa y coordinada de diferentes actores, gobiernos organizaciones de carácter civil, de esta manera la seguridad colectiva tiene que ser vista en términos de gobernanza de los riesgos globales, para ello es necesario abrir espacios en diferentes niveles, locales, nacionales, regionales, para que participen y debatan estos asuntos relacionados con la seguridad colectiva.

Determinar el marco y la participación es cuestión que permitirá devolver un protagonismo a NN. UU. por esencia de sus encorsetado e ineficaz papel que esta jugando en la actualidad, entre otras cuestiones por el bloqueo de fuerzas y Estados que se niegan a abandonar su papel dominante en el concierto internacional para dar paso a un mundo multipolar, de esta movilización deberían salir propuestas para unas NN. UU. que puedan jugar un papel importante en la construcción de una sociedad global mejor y mas segura, por establecer instituciones internacionales justas, representativas y legitimas que propicie condiciones sociales y económicas beneficiosas para toda la humanidad.

De esta manera dar una mayor eficacia y protagonismo a los programas dependientes de la Organización Mundial para la Salud, UNICEF, Programa de NN. UU. , para el desarrollo, la Organización Mundial delTrabajo, la UNESCO que hoy esta siendo cuestionados y atacados por quienes no aceptan un esquema multipolar d las relaciones internacionales.

En conclusión, repensar y modificar el sistema de Naciones Unidas enterrando el modelo derivado de la Guerra Fría y el reparto del Planeta en esferas de influencia de las grandes potencias es una cuestión vital no solo para responder eficazmente a las amenazas, riesgos y problemas globales, sino también para dotar a NN. UU. de una legitimad que hoy no tiene, para ello se señalan como cuestiones básicas el definir la Asamblea General como un poder legislativo internacional que este por encima de un Consejo de Seguridad y una Secretaria general, con poderes ejecutivos y el poder dotarse un Tribunal Universal, dejando en el aire el debate de la conveniencia o no de que las NNUU cuenten con una Fuerza Armada propia de carácter internacional al servicio directo de la Organización y contralado por la Asamblea General, asi como también es básico definir una serie de organismos adjuntos para desarrollar los diferentes programas aprobados por la Asamblea General, que terminen tanto con el FMI, como con el BM en su actual formulacion, funcionamiento y control por el gran capital.

Finalmente repetir que este esquema de replanteamiento del sistema de NNUU no puede llevarse a efecto desde un menoscabo de las distintas soberanías nacionales, ni mucho menos, del derecho de los pueblos a decidir libremente su sistema económico, social y cultural, dentro del respecto a la legalidad internacional, sino que tendría una función de coordinación de las acciones para trabajar por una orden internacional armonioso y una relaciones basadas en el muto beneficio que supere cualquier resto de colonialismo.

Desde estas perspectivas quienes defienden resolver la disyuntiva entre la construcción de un nuevo mundo o continuar la marcha hacia la barbarie destructiva del Planeta, desde una perspectiva favorable para el Planeta y para la mayoría de la humanidad tienen que ser conscientes de que este proceso tiene que conjugar la propuesta política, el debate académico con la capacidad para influir en la coyuntura internacional mediante una gran movilización popular de masas, porque sin la presión organizada de los Pueblos sera imposible que se pueda alcanzar un consenso internacional para afrontar un cambio real y profundo de las NN. UU. dando paso a un nuevo orden internacional porque resulta difícil creer que el eje atlántico Norte que ha dominado el orden internacional desde el derrumbe de la URSS vayan a aceptar su decadencia sin presentar batalla.

En este marcó tiene que ser la presión internacional de la sociedad civil quien reclame poner fin a un situación en la que el propio Secretario General de las Naciones Unidas reconoce que este Organismo no esta respondiendo como se necesita ante las múltiples crisis humanitarias, conflictos bélicos y emergencias médico-sanitarias que se sufren en todo el Planeta, y que por lo tanto de su transformación depende en gran medida que el futuro de la humanidad avance en Paz y desarrollo sostenible.

全球道德的基础
——国际贸易与中产阶级的兴起

克里斯托弗·瓦西洛普洛斯（Christopher Vasillopulos）*

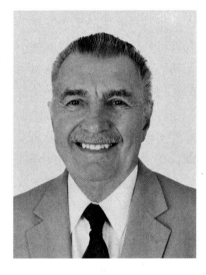

大约 2500 年前，在两个完全不同的地方，诞生了两位才智卓绝的人。他们沉着冷静，好思考，谨慎而又超然，尊重事实，对人性有着深刻的见解，不约而同地提出了一个问题：我该如何过这一生？他们的答案惊人的相似：以完善的自制为目标，高尚地生活（克己复礼）。

没有比这个更个人主义的答案了。因为责任的中心是个人，决定的核心也是个人。然而，正如孔子和亚里士多德所理解的那样，这个个体、这个潜在的完美的人，并不是他自己创造的，他独自生活也不合适，无论这种孤独沉思的生活有多么吸引他。或许，这个人比其他任何人都对他人负有责任，他也比其他任何人都更为清楚地认识到，如果不履行对他人的义务，他就无法完全实现自己的抱负。只有这样，他才能找到通往幸福、高尚地生活并自我完善的道路。

他首先要对自己的家庭负责，对与他共同生活的女人和她所生的孩子负责。正如他不能独善其身，他的家人也不能自我完善。一个家

---

* 克里斯托弗·瓦西洛普洛斯，美国东康涅狄格州立大学教授。

庭要想生存，就要同其他家庭共存。家庭之间需要合作，也需要规则来管理他们之间的合作与冲突。于是，在这一过程中，他们在几乎不知不觉中形成了一种社会秩序：社会。

但是，他们很快就得面对一个问题。如何能保证统治者不偏离道德的道路，他们怎样才能继续赢得人民的尊敬与顺从？孔子与亚里士多德对这几个问题有着不同的答案，这也反映出他们所处的不同社会。但是，必须记住的是，他们都相信，君主政体是政府的理想形式，只要君主是高尚的，并且体现了他所在社会的价值观。当然，问题依然存在。如何约束君主？他怎样才能像一个父亲对他的家庭服务那般，为他的人民效力呢？对孔子而言，建立一套教育体系，发现人才并将其培养成品德高尚的官员，至关重要。这些官员会受到规劝，在此过程中，下属会恭敬又不失分寸地提醒自己的上峰他可能偏离了正确的道路。与道德背道而驰的做法是危险的，因为它招致的是人民的反抗与绝望，是一个导致混乱的过程。

对亚里士多德而言，他也认为道德必不可少。规劝，虽不如孔子那样明确提倡，但也能从亚里士多德对悲剧的理解中推导出来。比如，在《安提戈涅》中，国王因不遵循神的律条而受到安提戈涅的规劝。虽然不如安提戈涅的规劝那么知名，但国王的儿子海蒙的规劝却更为重要，因为国王没有依照社会的利益来统治。虽然海蒙很懂分寸也不失对国王的尊敬，但他还是被无视了，于是灾难降临。在教育与规劝外，亚里士多德还提到了对绝对权力的制度制衡，以一种宪法秩序的形式，即贵族统治与民主政治的德性的谨慎结合。

我们这个时代的问题在本质上是一样的。如何寻找到并培养出一个为人民服务的统治者？21世纪的情况更为复杂。在这个迅速全球化的世界中，各国的统治者如何为人民服务？我认为，在贸易全球化的过程中或许能找到一些线索。想想看，数不清的国际交易以什么为前提：公平交易、尊重协议、诚实负责、重视长期关系而非短期牟取暴利，响应消费者与工人的需求与偏好。难道这些价值观同亚里士多德和孔子的实践智慧没有共通性吗？难道它们不是社会繁荣与稳定的物质基础吗？我想提出一些全球化的非物质后果。我认为，影响国际贸易的商业品德能有助于东、西方走到一起，通过在不同的文化与政治制度下建立相互尊重，而非仅仅依靠消除贫困与发展出数亿的中产阶级。全球交易的顺畅难道没有表明存在着一种深刻的、普遍的人性吗？被认为是诚实与相互尊重的公平交易，难道不是所有人际关系的基础吗？难道数以百万计的商贸交易不都在表明，尽管仍在竞争的舞台上，竞争对手们仍然相互合作以维持博弈的秩序吗？

我没有天真地以为所有民族国家都不得不面临的安全困境将会在大量的善意与商业成功中烟消云散。对抗竞争还将继续，往往还会因为猜疑与恐惧而加剧。未来永不确定，将会以越来越快的速度展开，并带来比以往都更为复杂的挑战，但同时也会带来更多的机遇。难道我们不能从新型冠状病毒大流行中吸取一些教训吗？人们可能希望在新一轮的疫情暴发中应对举措能更直截了当。没有哪个政府希望一场危机对其产生负面影响。不过，这种自我保护式的反应应尽量避免，因为太过关注自我形象而危及世界经济健康状况与良好的局势，这么做的风险太高。尽管疫情造成了诸多破坏，但它也激发出一些充满希望的变化。在美国，许多企业已经调整了自己的生产模式，以满足疫情期间的医疗需求。许多有竞争力的制药公司一直在合作，试图以最短的时间找到减轻症状的治疗方法与疫苗。我相信国际合作也是存在的。生活在纽约地区，我知道中国已经向美国运送了数以百万计的医疗防护设备。我相信美国也准备向世界各地运送数以千计的呼吸机。

这并不是在宣称国际紧张局势将会消失，也不意味着民族国家将不再以安全的名义谋求自身利益。完全有道德的国家比完全有道德的个人少见得多。不完美的人由不完美的官员所领导，有着不完美的社会秩序。然而，这种现实的评价不应蒙蔽我们的双眼，让我们看不到近五十年来的积极发展。当我还在加州大学伯克利分校攻读硕士学位的时候，没有人能想到中国会成为世界上第二大的成功经济体。也没有人会想到中国会比其他民族国家在世界范围内投资更多。更没有人会想到美中经济相互依赖，而世界的繁荣会依赖这一关系的滋长与丰富。谁也没有想到中国会诞生5亿中等收入群体。

最后，请允许我说明一点，经济上的相互依赖与中产阶层的兴起并不意味着东西方之间存在的深刻差异将会消失。但是，为了避免堕入各种形式的地狱，东西方必须就天堂的各种版本达成一致吗？为了避免自我毁灭的孤立，东西方就必须就正义与平等的含义达成一致吗？我意识到，相互依赖本身或许就是摩擦的一大来源。误会、沟通不畅总会时不时发生。交易越多，产生摩擦的几率就越高。尽管如此，明智的官员肯定会构思出冲突解决机制以确保繁荣与和平。在主要大国的领导下，各大国际组织能够得到加强，而各民族国家也能在一个相互尊重与赞赏的氛围中追求各自的利益。

当官员与领导人被引诱而偏离了德性的道路时，他们要记住，或有人应该提醒他们，他们到底有多依赖生产者。反过来，兢兢业业的中产阶层将不得不认识到，受法律约束、稳定、公平监管的政府对他们的繁荣是多么重要。全球化的前途在于从家庭、朋友、社会延伸到民族国家的德性，被孔子与亚里士多德如此看重的道德将延伸至全球社会。当各国领导人认识到其各自民族国家的成功取决于其他民族国家的成功时，各国之间的差异、对抗、激烈竞争，以及各国深刻的文化差异就不会导致战争。以公平交易与相互尊重所铺就的道德之路，可能永远也无法成为一条高速公路，但它却可能成为一条通往和平与繁荣的道路。（杨莉翻译）

原文：

The Basis of Global Virtue
—International Trade and Rising Middle Classes

Christopher Vasillopulos[*]

About 2500 years ago in two places, as different as they could be, two

---

* Christopher George Vasillopulos, prof. Eastern Connecticut State University.

brilliant men, calm, contemplative, prudent, detached, and respectful of the facts, each with a deep understanding of human nature, asked a profound question: how should I live? Their answers were remarkably similar: live virtuously by pursuing the goal of perfected self-mastery.

There could not have been a more individualistic answer. For the locus of responsibility was the individual. The locus of decision was the individual. Yet, as both Confucius and Aristotle understood, this individual man, this potentially perfect man, did not create himself. Nor was it proper for him to live alone, however a solitary contemplative life might appeal to him. Perhaps more than any other, this man had responsibilities to others. Perhaps more than any other, this man realized that he could not fulfill himself without fulfilling his duties to others. Only then could he find the path to happiness, to virtuous living, to self-perfection.

His first responsibility was to his family, to the woman he lived with and the children she bore. Just as he could not perfect himself alone, neither could his family. Families have to live with other families, if they are to survive. They need to cooperate; they need rules which govern their cooperation and their conflicts. They developed, almost without noticing, in the process a social order: society.

Almost immediately, a problem had to be confronted. How could the rulers be kept on the path of virtue, how could they continue to earn the respect and obedience of the people? Reflecting their different societies, Confucius and Aristotle had different answers to these questions. Yet, it must be remembered that both believed a monarchy was the ideal form of government, so long as the king was virtuous and so long as he embodied the values of his community. Of course, the problem remained. How could the king be controlled? How could he serve this people the way a father serves his family? For Confucius, a system of education that would find and train men to be virtuous officials was essential. These officials would be subject to remonstrance, a process by which subordinates would respectfully and tactfully remind an official that he might be straying from the proper path. Deviation from the path of virtue was dangerous, for it courted the disobedience and despair of the people, a process that would result in chaos.

For Aristotle, education for virtue was also considered essential. Remonstrance, although not as explicitly advocated as in Confucius, can be inferred from Aristotle's understanding of tragic plays. In Antigone, for example, the king is remonstrated by Antigone for not following divine rules. Less noted, but more important, the king was remonstrated by his son, Haemon for failing to rule in the community's interests. Though tactful and respectful, his son was ignored. Catastrophe resulted. To education and remonstrance Aristotle added institutional checks on absolute power, usually in the form of a constitutional order, one which would prudently mix the virtues of aristocracy and democracy.

The question for our time remains essentially the same. How can rulers befound and trained to serve their people? And in the twenty-first century a complication has been introduced. How can national rulers serve their people in a rapidly globalizing world? I believe clues might be found in the process of globalizing trade itself. Consider what millions of international exchanges presume: fair-dealing, respect for agreements, honesty, responsibility, the valuing of long term relations rather than short term profiteering, responsiveness to the needs and preferences of consumers and workers. Do not these values share the universe with the practical wisdom of Aristotle and Confucius? Do they not provide the material basis of prosperity and social stability? I should like to suggest some non-material consequences of globalization. I believe the commercial virtues which condition international trade can help bring East and West together, not simply by eliminating poverty and developing hundreds of millions of middle class people, but by building mutual respect despite differing cultures and political systems. Does not the very ease of global transactions indicate that there is a profound underlying universal human nature? Does not fair dealing, conceived of as honesty and mutual respect, the basis of all human relations? Do not millions of commercial exchanges indicate that while remaining in a competitive arena, rivals cooperate to keep the rules of the game in order?

I am not so naive as to presume that the security dilemma which must be confronted by all nation-states will dissolve in a sea of commercial success and good will. Rivalries will continue, often aggravated by suspicion and fear. Never certain, the future will unfold with increasing rapidity, bringing ever more complex challenges in its wake. But bringing as well, more possibilities. Are there not some lessons to be learned from the corona virus pandemic. One might hope that the response to new outbreaks would be more forthright. No government wants a crisis to reflect badly on it. However, this self-protective response must be avoided, for the stakes are too high to allow a concern for self-image to endanger the world's economic and physical health. For all its destruction, the pandemic has been stimulating some promising changes. In the U. S. many corporations have repurposed their manufacturing to meet the health needs of the crisis. Many competitive drug companies have been cooperating to find mitigating treatments and vaccines in record time. I believe there has been international cooperation as well. Living in the New York area, I am aware that China has shipped millions of health care protective devices to the U. S. I am certain that the U. S. is prepared to send thousands of ventilators around the world.

None is this is meant to claim that international tensions will disappear or that nation-states will not pursue their interests in the name of security. Completely virtuous nations are much rarer than completely virtuous individuals. Imperfect humans have imperfect social orders, led by imperfect officials. However, this realistic appraisal should not blind us to the positive developments of the last fifty or so years. When I was in graduate school at Berkeley, no one imagined that China would have the world's second most successful economy. No one imagined that China would be making more investments in the world that any other nation-state. No one imagined that the American and Chinese economies would be interdependent or that the prosperity of the world would depend on nurturing and enriching this relationship. No one imagined that there would be 500 million middle class Chinese citizens.

In conclusion, allow me to state that economic interdependence and rising middle classes do not mean that the profound differences between East and West will disappear. But do East and West have to agree on a version of heaven to avoid any version of hell? Do East and West have to agree on what Justice or Equality mean to avoid self-destructive isolation? I realize that interdependence itself might be a source of friction. Misunderstandings, miscommunication will occur from time to time. The more transactions the more chances for friction. However, intelligent officials can certainly devise conflict resolution mechanisms that will insure prosperity and peace. International organizations can be strengthened while China and U. S. pursues its interest in an atmosphere of mutual respect and appreciation.

As officials and leaders are tempted to deviate from the path of virtue, they will have to remember or be reminded how dependent they are on the productive classes. In turn the hard-working middle classes will have to appreciate how essential law-bound, stable, fairly administered government is to their prosperity. The promise of globalization is that the extension of virtuous from family, friends, community, to nation-state, so valued by Confucius and Aristotle, will extend to the global community. When it is appreciated by leaders that the success of their nation-state depends on the success of other nation-states, their differences, their rivalries, their intense competition, along with their profound cultural differences, will not descend to war. The path to virtue, paved with fair-dealing and mutual respect, may never be a highway, but it may become a road to peace and prosperity.

塑造国际关系的新范式

威廉·琼斯（William Jones）[*]

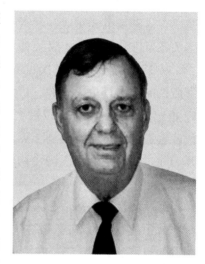

如果说全世界从这场新冠肺炎疫情的惨痛经历中汲取了什么教训的话，那一定是各国必须合作才能确保自身的生存。病毒不分国界，不分种族和信仰，不讲阶级和地位，传播起来毫不留情。全世界都面临威胁。当所有国家都被疫情的突然暴发与其严重程度所震惊时，中国政府对武汉疫情迅速而彻底的应对，为其他多数国家试图在本国遏制疫情的蔓延设立了典范。中国积极向许多疫情国家提供医疗设备，输送医护人员，同时还为他国利用中国经验抗击疫情尽了一份力。

中国的援助唯独漏了美国。并不是中国没有向美国伸出援手，中国多半这么做了，但特朗普政府并不愿意接受来自中国的帮助。当新型冠状病毒终于引起美国重视时，美中关系正处于非常低迷的状态。特朗普总统挑起了贸易摩擦，而一些美国政策精英则担心，中国崛起成为全球经济增长的主要引擎，正在影响美国单方面为世界制定规则的能力，这种担心已经到了完全偏执的程度。特朗普政府没有就中国对全球治理中美国这一"单边"角色的关切去调整适应，却似乎着

---

* 威廉·琼斯，美国《全球策略信息》杂志华盛顿分社社长。

手破坏中国经济增长并在全世界面前抹黑中国的政策。

但特朗普没能采取中国成功遏制武汉疫情的一系列措施，无疑是导致美国死亡人数激增的原因之一。意识到这一失职可能导致他在11月的选举中落败，现在他听从了自己新保守主义顾问的建议，"谴责"中国据说没有更早地向美国通报疫情的严重性。因此，世界上两个最重要的国家之间正朝着出现裂痕的方向前进。

这种进退两难的局面清楚地表明，我们称作"地缘政治"的政治前景已不能再成为国与国关系的主导心态了。坚持零和博弈的地缘政治思维只能导致冲突，甚至战争。我们需要的是一种国与国关系的新范式，这种新范式可以在习近平主席所说的大国关系中找到。这一大国关系牵涉哪些方面？又要如何建立？

从17世纪末到第二次世界大战结束，世界历史在很大程度上是由所谓的大国竞争决定的。1763年，七年战争以英国的胜利而告终，17世纪法兰西的主导地位被大不列颠所取代。然后直到19世纪70年代，崛起的德意志威胁到了英国在欧洲的霸权。为了对抗德国，英国开始通过英、法、俄三国协约对德国进行包围。这导致了第一次世界大战。

第一次世界大战后，人们就有了这样一种共识：多国之间长达数年的战争成本太过高昂，需要找到另外一种解决办法。威尔逊总统试图以他自己的方式，在他对国际联盟的提议中找到一个解决方案。然而，胜利的一方，英国和法国对惩罚德国——他们所谓的侵略国更感兴趣，于是，随着1919年报复性的《凡尔赛条约》的通过，国家联盟成为一纸空文，而这一决定也为一场新的战争埋下了种子。

第二次世界大战后，曾作为威尔逊政府的一员，并在第一次世界大战期间目睹了国际联盟失败的富兰克林·罗斯福，认为需要作出新的努力来建立这样一个机构。在他的努力下，联合国成立了，并自此之后成为全世界国家汇聚一堂、通过外交而非战争来解决他们不满的首要论坛。而美国，作为唯一一个经济没有遭到战争严重破坏的国家，成为重建世界经济的主要力量。罗斯福的目标是将全世界联系在一起，让包括英国在内的所有帝国消失，并开启非洲与亚洲的工业化进程。他还希望在美国、中国、苏联与英国之间建立某种"大国关系"，以维护世界的稳定，预防冲突。但随着罗斯福的过世，温斯顿·丘吉尔开始重塑美国的政策以恢复"大国政治"的概念，把美国卷入其中成为"执法者"，以削弱苏联的影响力。渐渐地，罗斯福的愿景被搁置一旁，美国政策在很大程度上由采用了丘吉尔帝国主义观点的"英美派别"所主导。约翰·F.肯尼迪试图恢复罗斯福的部分愿景，但却在努力中遭到了杀害。

随着1991年苏联解体，美国凭借其在北约组织与七国集团中的主导地位，成为世界政治中类似于唯一"规则制定者"的存在。事实证明，虽然这些"规则"并没有给世界大多数国家带来多大的好处，几场重大的金融危机、持续不断的军事冲突以及第三世界一直处于发展不充分状态都证明了这一点，但这却给予了美国一个独特的地位，一个英美派众人都不准备放弃的地位，包括大多数特朗普总统的顾问在内。如今，与中国日益加剧的对峙，就是他们不愿在世界面临可怕流行病时分享权力的最好例证。

但这一地位将很难维持。尽管特朗普总统有意召开七国集团会议，毫无疑问是为了将其"盟友"拽进他对中国的"谴责游戏"里，但七国集团的领导人不太可能对这样的行动表现出极大的热情。他们中的不少人已经同中国建立起了相当友好的工作关系，一些人对特朗普总统"美国优先"的政策也相当不满。而所有人都清楚地认识到中国在世界经济中发挥的重要作用。事实上，不少国家都从中国的"一带一路"倡议中获益良多。大家也清楚地认识到，如果没有中国的合作，新型冠状病毒引发的大动荡很可能导致新的大萧条，所有国家都会遭受巨大损失。

即使是在美国国内，也有人明白这种反华势头将会损害美国，美国人并没有完全忘记罗斯福总统的传统。如果特朗普总统拿"谴责中国"当他的竞选口号的话，他可能严重低估了美国选民识破这种雕虫小技的能力——试图掩盖其政府在这场阻止新型冠状病毒在美传播的战役中真正的政策错误的伎俩。

在当前形势下，实现中美大国关系不是一件容易的事。但这种关系的原则是既有的。甚至早在"大国政治"时代之前，我们就曾于1648年签署了《威斯特伐利亚和约》，结束了长达三十年的那场完全摧毁了西欧的战争。《威斯特伐利亚和约》基于的原则是"对方的利益"。这就意味着，参与缔约的各方必须考虑到对方可能得到的利益，并将之纳入协议。《威斯特伐利亚和约》即习近平主席所称之"双赢局面"。

此时此刻，特朗普政府无意在涉及中国的问题上关注"对方的利益"。毫无疑问，蓬佩奥等人将会敲锣打鼓地试图鼓动美国人民及其盟友加入他们对北京的讨伐当中。不过，尽管呼声甚高，但恐怕不会有太多人投身其中，甚至不会有太多美国选民支持这项徒劳无益、适得其反的事业。为了如此危险的尝试"集结军队"失败的话，甚至会迫使总统寻找一条不同的道路，因为当前选择的这条路前面是个死胡同。（杨莉翻译）

原文：

Shaping a New Paradigm in International Relations

William Jones[*]

If there is anything the world has learned from the traumatic experience of the coronavirus pandemic it is that countries must cooperate in order to assure their own survival. The virus knows no borders, does not distinguish between races or creeds, and moves relentlessly with no respect for class or status. The threat is universal. While all countries were taken by surprise by the suddenness and the virulence of the outbreak, the rapid and most thor-

---

* William Jones, Chief, *Executive Intelligence Review*, Washington Bureau.

ough response by the Chinese government to the outbreak in Wuhan served as a model that most other countries attempted to implement in stemming the spread in their own regions. China's pro-active outreach with medical equipment and personnel to many of the stricken countries, also contributed in helping them use the knowledge gained by China in their own anti-epidemic efforts.

The lone exception to this help was the United States. Not that China didn't offer such help. They probably did. But the Trump Administration was not willing to accept help from China. By the time the coronavirus made itself felt in the United States, US-Chinese relations were at a very low ebb. President Trump's "trade friction" and the fear of some in the U. S. policy elites that China's rise, as the major engine of global growth, was affecting the power of the U. S. to unilaterally "set the rules" for the world, had reached the stage of outright paranoia. Rather than accommodate China's concerns about this "unilateral" role of the United States in global governance, the Trump Administration now seems embarked on a policy of undermining the growth of the Chinese economy and discrediting China in the eyes of the world.

But the failure of President Trump to adopt the string of measures China successfully used to quell the epidemic in Wuhan, no doubt contributed to the overwhelming number of deaths in the U. S. In his awareness that this failure could lead to his defeat in November, he has now followed the advice of his neoconservative advisers to "blame China" for allegedly not informing the U. S. about the seriousness of the disease earlier. As a result, we are moving in the direction of a major rift between the two most important nations in the world.

This dilemma clearly shows that the political outlook of what we call "geopolitics" can no longer remain the dominant mind-set in relations between nations. Sticking to the geopolitical mindset of the zero-sum game can only lead to conflict, and even war. What is required is a new paradigm of relations between nations. Such a paradigm can be found in what President

Xi calls a major-power relationship. What does this entail? And how can this be established?

From the end of the 17th century until the end of World War Ⅱ, world history was largely determined by what "Great Power competition." The dominant role of France in the 17th century was replaced by Great Britain after the British victory in the Seven Year's War in 1763. Then by the 1870s, a rising Germany threatened the British hegemony in Europe. To counter that Great Britain began an encirclement of Germany through the Triple Entente of Great Britain, France and Russia. This led to World War I.

After the World War I, there was something of an understanding that the age of wars between nations bore such a heavy cost that an alternative had to be found. President Wilson attempted, in his own way, to find such a solution in his proposal for the League of Nations. But the victorious powers, Great Britain and France, were more interested in punishing Germany, the country they claimed to be the aggressor, and a League of Nations became something of a dead letter with the passage of the vindictive Versailles Treaty in 1919, a decision that planted seeds of a new war.

After the World War Ⅱ, Franklin Roosevelt, who had witnessed the failure of the United Nations as a member of the Wilson government during World War I, felt that a new effort was needed to create such a body. From his efforts came the United Nations, which has since served as the premier forum for all nations of the world to come together to resolve their grievances through diplomacy rather than war. While the United States, as the only country whose economy had not been seriously damaged by the war, became the primary source for rebuilding the world economy, Roosevelt's goal was to bring the world together, to dissolve all empires, even the British, and to begin a process of industrializing Africa and Asia. He also wanted to craft something of a "major-power relationship" between the U. S., China, the Soviet Union and Great Britain to maintain stability and prevent conflict in the world. But with the death of Roosevelt, Winston Churchill began to reshape U. S. policy in order to restore the notion of "Great Power politics" bringing the United States in as the "enforcer" and directed at undermining the influence of the Soviet Union. More and more, the Roosevelt vision was brushed aside, and U. S. policy became largely dominated by an "Anglo-American faction," which had adopted Churchill's Imperialist viewpoint. John F. Kennedy tried to restore some of the Roosevelt vision, but was killed in the effort.

With the demise of the Soviet Union in 1989, the U. S. , through its dominant position in the G-7 and in NATO, became something of the sole "rule-maker" in world politics. And while those "rules" have not proven terribly beneficial to most of the world, as is witnessed by the major financial crises, the continuous military conflicts, and continued underdevelopment in the Third World, it gave the United States a unique position which the Anglo-American crowd is not prepared to forego, including most of President Trump's advisers. And the growing face-off with China today is a prime example of their unwillingness to share power in a world now facing a dreadful pandemic.

But it is a position that will be hard to sustain. While President Trump is intent on calling a G7 meeting, no doubt with the intention of bringing his "allies" on board his China "blame game," it is highly unlikely that G7 leaders will be terribly enthusiastic about such a campaign. Many of them have established a rather cordial working relationship with China. Some of them are not terribly happy with President Trump's "America First" policy. And all of them are clearly aware of the major role China is playing in the world economy. Indeed, many of these countries have benefited greatly from China's Belt and Road Initiative. There is also a clear understanding that without China's cooperation, the turmoil caused by the coronavirus could well lead to a new great depression in which all nations will suffer greatly.

Even within the United States there are those who understand that this anti-China thrust will damage the U. S. , and the FDR tradition has not been completely forgotten by Americans. And if President Trump is prepared to use "Blame China" as his election campaign slogan, he may have seriously underestimated the ability of the American voters to see through such a cheap ploy to hide the real policy mistakes of his own Administration in the fight to stop the spread of COVID-19 in the U. S.

In the present situation, achieving a major-power relationship between China and the U. S. will not be an easy task. But the principles of such a relationship are readily at hand. Even before the era of "great power politics," we had in 1648 the Peace of Westphalia, which ended a thirty-year period of war, which totally devastated western Europe. The principle on which that Peace was based on "the good of the other. " That meant that the parties engaged in creating the peace had to also take consideration to the benefit that would be had by the opposite party and to incorporate that into the agreement. Westphalia was what President Xi would call a "win-win situation. "

At the moment, the Trump Administration has no interest in focusing on "the good of the other" with regard to China. And Pompeo and others will no doubt beat the drums to try and mobilize the American people and their allies to join them in their crusade against Beijing. But it's unlikely, in spite of all the shouting, that there will be a big turn out for this crusade, and there may not even be a great deal of support among American voters for such a futile and self-defeating cause. And the failure to "rally the troops" around such a dangerous endeavor may even force the President to find a different path, as the one presently chosen will lead to a total dead end.

"新冠病毒肺炎"危机

——风险抑或机遇?

扎哈里·扎哈里耶夫 (Zahari Mihaylov Zahariev)[*]

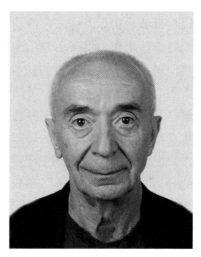

　　近来,在这个星球的词汇中几乎没有任何一个概念能比"危机"一词更扎眼了。它出现在每一篇政治声明的开头和结尾,衡量着一切经济与政治的预测。它颠覆了所有传统的日常惯例,对近来那些难以反驳的观点进行反思,在社会、政治、经济,甚至法定的固有社会标准中处处布雷。而所有这一切都是由一场疫情引发的。很自然的,问题来了:尽管有所变异但开端却广为人知的病毒,比如"新型冠状病毒",是否可能在短短几个月的时间里颠覆整个世界?一个单一的、无论有多严重的流行病是否有可能在一个包罗万象的毁灭性结构范围内引发海啸般的危机?

　　要回答这些问题,其前提是要接受一些不同的,甚至时常相互排斥的设想。而真相,其实简单得多。"新冠病毒肺炎"不过揭开了公共关系各领域内长期潜藏的危机进程的面纱——从日益加剧的社会不平衡与医疗体系难以满足公共需求,到毁掉了国家作为公共利益平衡器的市场自由主义,到威胁了地缘政治稳定、不断深化的地缘政治层

---

　　* 扎哈里·扎哈里耶夫,保加利亚"一带一路"全国联合会主席。

级的结构性转移，再到经济安全，最后也是最重要的地球生态平衡。然而，无论这些发展中的"绊脚石"在这场危机中的表现乍一看有多么不一样，它们都有着一个相同的根源。也即是说，现存的社会关系已经触及了其文明程度可达到的极限。人类正迈入历史发展的新阶段，但还不确定要以何种方式进入，而历史发展新阶段必然需要一种新的社会契约。资本主义已经完全耗尽了它的历史资源，而新自由主义，无论其表现为何种形式，实际上也已是穷途末路：但历史本身并没有终结，这不过是文明发展篇章中的一页翻过去了而已。

所有这一切都导向了一场日益尖锐的对抗，一边是社会变革的客观需求，一边是同大国利益联系在一起、绵延了几个世纪的现状。新冠病毒肺炎实际上标志着推动这两大的力量间的公开冲突。统治精英们对全球化作为发展引擎的态度发生了急剧转变。"全球问题需要全球应对"这一过渡阶段的基本信条越来越难以符合他们唯利是图的权力野心设下的狭小限制。帝国主义又回到了它的起点——民族国家的堡垒。这些又助长了另一种流行病——种族与种族文化的对立、沙文主义与排外主义、种族主义与国家的排他性。

因此，尽管当前形势还存在各种不确定，但有一样却是肯定的——"新冠病毒肺炎"不仅标志着我们未来社会、文化与政治生活出现了转折点，同时，对国际关系、对所有国际共同体、整个全球经济网络以及那些或多或少都支撑了全球安全的政治机构而言，它也标志着转折点的出现。受这场流行病危机所驱动，经济发展进程又助推了新的地缘战略与地缘政治灾难。其中，有三个尤其令人不安的趋势。

趋势一，南北半球的新分歧。全球经济受到冲击，产量急剧下降，在某些行业，产量几已降至零水平。供应受阻与外贸机制又加剧了这些问题。大规模隔离使得消费锐减。世界要为两位数的负增长做好准备。随着失业人数的不断增加，这还意味着对流行性疾病的恐惧很快就会被饥饿引发的恐惧所取代，而饥饿会导致数百万人流落街头。不过，正如德国分析家彼得斯（Stefan Peters）指出的那样，"北半球的经济危机最多只能导致一场严重的流感，南半球的国家感受到的才是经济衰退的冲击。商品价格的骤降与旅游业的衰落，以及来自移民工人汇款的减少，已经导致了不少南半球国家的外汇与政府收入的崩塌"。因此，我们不难预测，随着疫情即将触顶，尤其是在非洲与拉丁美洲触顶，极端贫困、不稳定、政治镇压与暴力犯罪将急剧增加。由此造成的混乱又将导致新的移民浪潮冲击日益自我孤立的北半球。

趋势二是全球政治中多中心主义将进一步发展。中国与俄罗斯的经济及地缘政治地位的加强，两国与许多中亚、东南亚国家，以及诸如印度、南非与巴西等能源大国之间一体化联系的日益加强，都导致了世界政治正日益形成新的全球利益极点。在这一点上，中国的角色尤其重要。"命运共同体"的理念，与其相关的"一带一路"倡议正让中国在历史发展阶段中处于"火车头"的地位。中国成功抗击疫情，其经济的迅速复苏，都极大地增强了其作为全球经济增长主要驱动力的可信度，特别是经济迅速复苏这一点，对许多国家及跨国公司的经济生活而言是十分关键的一个因素。同样，对于人类寻找 21 世纪发展的新视野而言，也十分关键。正如美国国家情报委员会（the US National Intelligence Council）最新的报告《全球趋势 2025：转型的世界》（*Global Trends 2025：A Transformed World*）指出的那样，"中国将在世界经济中处于领先地位，并将决定财富和经济影响力自西向东转移"。

趋势三是由美国与北约组织日益加剧的军事与政治对抗所决定的。除了传统的军事冲突形式外，军事经济对抗也越来越多地出现在前沿，从而缩短了从传统的军事威胁发展为毁灭性的全球冲突的路径。这种侵略手段的主要工具之一便是所谓的混合战争中出现的多种多样的非常规手段——对他国的信息资源进行渗透，制造恐慌，为有目的地建立起来的政治实体与社会团体提供资金资助，在网络上进行大规模的虚假信息宣传，等等。

这种仇恨政策的一大关键因素便是新自由主义大师米尔顿·弗里德曼（Milton Friedman）提出的"休克主义"——通过战争、恐怖主义行动，自然灾害或类似的群体性冲击，来扰乱公众基本导向，以便强制实施不受欢迎的经济、政治举措。在他看来，混乱与方向迷失应该被用来达成这一目标，并在引发的危机中采取"休克疗法"。

所有这些工具如今都用在了一场自冷战以来前所未有的针对中国、俄罗斯及每一个反对美国于 1990 年确立的单极世界现状的国家的仇恨运动中。这场混合战争的武器中再次出现了意识形态与宗教不宽容的手段，全民反对及仇外心理，这是极其危险的。继反犹太主义病毒后，反俄主义、反中主义病毒又开始在今天的信息与宣传领域内登场。

尽管如此，这些进程的消极发展到目前为止还不能决定当前文明发展危机的最终结果。向前发展的抵抗力量正取得进展。公共利益促进并加强了公民意志，并日益凸显出公民意志的国际性。这一点，再加上成功得到巩固的两极地缘政治现状，肯定会激发人们的乐观情绪，这场围绕"新冠病毒肺炎"大流行的结构性动荡，也可能成为一个新的、更好的全球思考与行动的开端，以建立一个更安全、更公正的世界。毕竟，中文的"危机"一词是"危"（代表危险）与"机"（意为机遇）两字的组合，是危险与机遇两种概念的结合。（杨莉翻译）

原文：

The "COVID-19" Crisis
—Risk Or Chance?

Zahari Mihaylov Zahariev*

There is hardly a concept that has lately been more evident in the planet's glossary than the word "crisis". It is at the beginning and end of

* Zahari Mihaylov Zahariev, President, Bulgaria National Association for the Belt and Road.

every political statement, measuring all economic and political projections. It reverses the old-fashioned daily routine, rethinks difficult-to-contest recent views, "mines" social, political, economic and even statutory fixed social standards. And all this, provoked by an endemic flu situation. The question naturally arises: Is it possible for a mutating, but nevertheless well-known in its genesisvirus, such as "COVID-19", to overturn the entire social universe in just a few months? Is it possible for a single, however serious be it, health pandemic, to whirl a tsunami crisis with such an all-embracing destructive structural scope?

The truth, which is very common in such situations, "COVID-19" only lifted the veil that hides long-running crisis processes in all spheres of public relations-from growing social imbalances and the inability of the healthcare system to meet public needs, through market liberalism that is ruining the state as a balancer of public interests, to the deepening tectonic shifts of geopolitical strata that threaten geopolitical stability, to economic security, and last but not least, to the planet's ecological balance. However, all these "stumbling blocks" in development, however different be they at first glance in their crisis expression, have one root in common. And it is that existing social relations have reached the limit of their civilizational adequacy. The new phase of historical development in the approaches towards which humanity is uncertainly heading, definitely requires a new social contract. Capitalism has completely exhausted its historical resource, and neoliberalism, in all its manifestations, is indeed the end: But not of history itself, but only of one of the pages that civilization unfolds.

All this leads to an increasingly sharp confrontation between objectively needed social change and the status quo associated with dominant for centuries power interests. The coronavirus pandemic has actually signaled an open clash between the forces driving these two trends. Hence the sharp turn in the attitude of the ruling elites towards globalization as an engine of development. The basic credo in the transition period, that "global problems require global responses", is increasingly difficult to fit within the narrow limits of their venal power ambitions. Imperialism goes back to its beginning-the cita-del of the nation-state. All of this feeds another pandemic—that of ethnic and ethno-cultural opposition, of chauvinism and xenophobia, of racism and na-tional exclusivity.

Therefore, with all the uncertainty of the situation, we can definitely say one thing— "COVID-19" marks not only a turning point for our future social, cultural and political life, but also for international relations, for all integration communities and for the whole global network of economic and political institutions which more or less support global security. The economic processes, driven by the pandemic crisis, propel new geostrategic and geo-political disasters. Among them are three particularly troubling trends.

The first is a new divide between the Global North and the Global South. The global economy is in shock. Production is sharply decreasing and in some sectors it is reduced to near zero. The problems are exacerbated by the blocked supply and foreign trade system. Mass isolation sharply reduces consumption. The world is preparing for double-digit negative growth. Along with the increasing number of unemployed people, this suggests that fears from the pandemic will soon give way to starvation that can bring millions to the streets. But as German analyst Stefan Peters notes "nevertheless the eco-nomic crisis in the global North will result in, at most, a severe flu. The brunt of economic downturn will be felt by the countries of the global South. The drastic decline in commodity prices and tourism, as well as the decline in remittances from migrant workers, is already causing a collapse in the government and foreign exchange revenues of many of these countries. " Therefore, it is not difficult to predict that with the imminent peak of the dis-ease, especially in Africa and Latin America, extreme poverty, instability, political repression and criminal violence will increase sharply. The chaos thus created will send new waves of emigrants storming the increasingly self-isolated global North.

The second is that of increasing polycentrism in global politics. The strengthening economic and geopolitical positions of China and Russia and the growing integrative ties between them, many Central and Southeast Asian countries and resource giants such as India, South Africa and Brazil, are increasingly shaping a new pole of global interests in world politics. Of particular importance in this respect is China's role. The philosophy of the "shared future" and the related "the Belt and Road" Initiative have propelled the PRC in a position of locomotive in historical development. China's successful battle with the epidemic and the rapid recovery of its economy, which is an important key factor in the economic life of many countries and multinational companies, has tremendously strengthened its credibility as a major driver of global economic growth. But also in the search for new horizons for the development of humanity in the 21st century. As noted in the most recent report by the US National Intelligence Council "Global Trends 2025: A Transformed World" China will have a leading position in the world economy and will predetermine the "transfer of wealth and economic influence from West to East".

The third trend is determined by the growing military-political confrontation caused by the US and NATO. Alongside the traditional forms of military conflict, military-economic confrontation is increasingly emerging in the forefront, shortening the path from the traditional military threat to a devastating global conflict. A major tool in this aggressive approach is the rich arsenal of unconventional means of the so-called hybrid war-infiltration of the information resources of other countries, inciting panic, financing of purposefully created political entities and social formations, massive disinformation campaign on the web, etc.

A key factor in this hatred policy is the "doctrine of shock", launched by neo-liberalism guru Milton Friedman-forming public disorientation through collective shocks from wars, acts of terrorism, natural disasters and similar, in order to impose unpopular economic and political measures. In his view, chaos and disorientation should be used to make this happen and to use "shock therapy" in the created crisis situation.

All of these tools are being deployed today in an unprecedented since the Cold War campaign of hatred against China, Russia, and every country opposing the unipolar status quo affirmed by the United States in 1990. It is extremely dangerous that in the arsenal of this hybrid war reappeared the instruments of ideological and religious intolerance, xenophobia and national opposition. After the virus of anti-Semitism, those of anti-Russism and anti-Chinism began to swirl on the information and propaganda scene today.

The negative development of these processes, however, does not by far determine the outcome of the current crisis of civilizational development. The resistance forces of progress are gaining ground. Public interests stimulate and strengthen the civil will, giving it an increasingly prominent international character. And this, coupled with the successfully consolidating bipolar geopolitical status quo, certainly inspires optimism that the structural turmoil surrounding the "COVID-19" pandemic could also be a new, better start to global thinking and global action for a safer and more just world. After all the Chinese hieroglyph for crisis combines the notion of "danger", respectively "risk" and the concept of "opportunity", respectively "chance".

后新冠肺炎疫情世界的
经济、权力与安全

苏莱曼·森索伊（Süleyman Şensoy）*

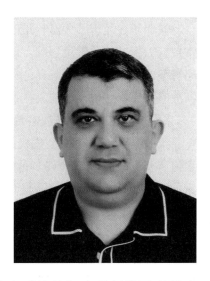

　　2019 年 12 月新型冠状病毒被鉴定为"COVID-19"之后，世卫组织宣布该病毒在全球范围的暴发为"大流行"。国际舞台面临意想不到的危机。

　　在过去 12 年中，土耳其亚洲战略研究中心在众多报告中提出的宏观及部门"战略转型"建议和风险分析并未在土耳其及共享这些信息的国家的公共、私人和民间社会得到足够重视，而不断发展的新冠病毒肺炎大流行则首次确证了这些建议和分析。随着大流行的加剧，对权力和财产模型（这一模型已被安全和国防生态系统的加速受创等因素所改变）的及时捕获变得更加困难。

　　全球治理在平衡技术、经济、军事和政治威胁的同时，大流行使所有行为者措手不及。在国际舞台上，确保生命安全已被提上世界议事日程之首，而当市场、国际贸易和国家间交通被暂停之时，许多国家的基础设施和经济却显露出不足。这一全球大流行给那些将卫生系统等软性区域排在次要位置的大国一个教训。至于疫情将持续多久、疫苗研究及其可能出现的副作用等不可预测的情况，则需要时间来估

---

* 苏莱曼·森索伊，土耳其亚洲战略研究中心主席。

量并始终拥有对应的最新方案。在当前和未来对大流行病的预测中，许多国家缺乏经济和政治战略/基础设施，这是全球危机带来的变化和转型的先兆。

对于每个未失去基础设施控制权的国家，"控制治理"的概念似乎是其基本范例。无论下一病毒名称如何或危机如何复杂，当前的流行病都是一所全球性学校，人们应当汲取教训，来保护经济、社会和安全基础设施。由于我们清楚各国因死亡造成的人口减少带来的巨大风险，因此更应关注重症监护、插管和死亡人数，而不是病例数。减少损失是面对坏事的最佳选择。同样，食物、水和卫生安全已成为各国和全球治理的首要任务和合作领域。

我们正在经历的大流行是改变生产、消费、增长和包含安全在内的常规权力标准的关键里程碑。现在，对国家和国际免疫系统、方案和战略转型的准备进行重新解释已成为当务之急。在这种情况下，土耳其亚洲战略研究中心很早以前就在最高级别上主动向本国及许多国家提出的"未来安全生态系统及其战略转型"，已成为各国的优先事项。

很难预测下一个复杂危机的发生地区或大爆发将是什么。当前的大流行折射出：在世界许多地方，对安全的威胁不太可能来自其他国家的军队，而是源于一系列问题，例如经济崩溃、政治压迫、饥荒、人口过度增长、种族分裂、战争、内部冲突、区域和国家冲突、破坏自然环境、恐怖主义、有组织犯罪、政府针对其本国人民的暴力行为、"流行病"、危险品、偷运人口、武器和毒品贩运、洗钱、旨在破坏新兴民主国家市场稳定的大规模金融欺诈。

2007—2008 年的国际金融危机，2011 年美国的"占领华尔街"抗议，伦敦、法兰克福和巴黎的学生和激进主义者抗议，西亚北非政治动荡以及在撒哈拉以南非洲和东亚发生的人道主义危机；关于法律和政治、安全与自由、民粹主义、多元主义和民主，宗教、种族、阶级、人种和少数民族的断层线以及大流行（主要包括西方国家）的辩论变得更加脆弱。

随着病毒对整个世界影响的迅速增强，在讨论国际组织的有效性、不足和变化时，人们将目光投向了各国的经济状况。为了减轻危机的影响，使公共债务、私人债务和家庭债务同时上升到新高度的强制性和优惠性的终结，是无法控制的。此外，许多受这些指标约束的国家将谈不上政治独立甚至维持稳定。

在讨论世卫组织、国际货币基金组织和欧盟等国际组织如何有益于全球体系时，这种有效威慑的出现应该是所有国家首先要质疑的因素之一。在新的国际秩序和安全条例中，国家和全球能力之间的联盟和差异，而非传统的政党，将决定动荡的严重性和持续时间。在这种情况下，为了定义新的地缘政治，有义务研究以前从未使用过的公式。在"微观民族主义""一体化"和"不可预测性"框架内形成的国际秩序和制度的未来，取决于由"权力与正义"支撑的世界观。

土地最有价值的时期是"帝国时代"，随着"工业革命"的出现，机器变得更有价值。毕竟，民族国家诞生了，我们今天的"信息时代"是一个促进"微观民族主义"的国际体系。可以毫不夸张地预言，大流行会加速对此事的有力确认。还应强调的是，"微观民族主义"与种族无关（即使团结在加密货币周围的人士也可以包括在内），任何组织上的差异都可以看作是微观民族主义。

正是"批判思想"和"功绩"为新时代的成功竞争提供了基本规则。实际上，必须通过重新解释这些参数来揭示"制度基础设施"的力量，这些参数在当今环境下已成为整个世界历史的参考。此外，在世界文明僵局这一点上，对于第二次世界大战后（在与今天相比高度理想的条件下）建立的国际体系，需要在"权力与正义"的基础上重新加以解释。否则，不太可能提及可管理的世界或国家的状况。为了支持这种"制度基础设施"，管理不可预测性和冲突的专业领域（即使它是通过处理实践中的危机而发展起来的）也需要更加有意识地以虚拟方式进一步发展。

正如我们多年来所说的那样，"权力和权力所有权"的概念正在迅速变化。传统的一切都会被改变，尤其是大规模军队、大规模人群、大规模公务员和专家。这种大流行将进一步提高国防工业能力或其支撑机构（包括生产企业）的变化率。显然，在信息甚于货币更体现价值的时期，需要不断更新对新传统的需求。在这种情况下，世界正在进入一个传统积累的市场价值迅速熔化的时期。对人们而言可能是房子、车子或投资工具，对国家而言就是军队。在新的权力分配中，决定性的是将重点放在新传统是什么、其经济对应是什么以及应该如何转变。

在被新冠肺炎疫情改变后的商业模式中，跟踪并加深由生产放缓而释放出的生态气息，将确保这场危机带来的重要机会不被浪费。同样，"预期管理"能力将能够控制社会各阶层在大流行中的多维创伤，这将是公共行政部门社会经济安全的关键。

对于所有国家而言，按传统发展自己的基础设施来解决国家间体系中可能出现的问题，并不断改善其建立在经济、军事等基础上的优势，在大流行中失去了重要性。高失业率国家和经济脆弱的国家都在努力应对由于病毒引起的制度性和体系化基础设施崩溃的威胁。

昨天有价值的信息和知识能否在未来甚至今天保持其价值还不得而知。在如此动荡的时刻，至关重要的是在国家中长期计划中制定关键战略。

在全球经济中，除了当前的新型冠状病毒之外，还可以预见在后新冠肺炎疫情时期将持续的经济停滞。人们认为，收缩的影响将是持久的，经济收缩将在国家、区域和全球范围内发生。预测显示，2020年全球经济将萎缩4%—5%。据称，全球经济所处的这种停滞和下降水平，将导致国际资本资产和产能有限的生产投资的停滞，并使外国子公司资本缩水。

在这种情况下，制度基础设施和风险管理似乎不足以抵御这种不利情况，因后者会带来更多的行业停滞不前，例如首当其冲的制造业、房地产、商业和管理活动，批发和零售贸易、汽车和物流，运输、储存和通信，住宿和餐饮服务，艺术、表演以及娱乐等服务。

当前的萎缩和衰退也有可能使全球暂时免于战争，并可能使人们从"债务—金钱—债务"的螺旋式资源危机中得到喘息。但是在这种情况下，债务和资本分配中的相对福利分担将继续使人们的处境不可置信地恶化。

根据经济学家最近的评估，全球经济由于此次大流行估计将遭受约5.5万亿美元的打击。衍生品市场的损失已达数十万亿美元，面临失业风险的人数已接近10亿。据估计，大流行对发达国家经济造成的损失将超过1929年、1975年、2008—2009年衰退的水平。在预测中，只有在2023年才会恢复疫情之前的经济水平。

全球商业模式、权力和财产分配、安全与国防，都会被由大流行再次确证的核心领域如"机器人""生物技术""人工智能""纳米技术""空间"和"战略服务"所改变。危机再次使过去15年来一直表达的新战略环境中"安全"和"权力"的概念为人所知。这种情况要求在国防、安全、外交和社会经济领域运作的制度及其利益相关者通过重新解释这些新的传统概念来重新组织。在这种情况下，各国最重要的认识是，无须里里外外寻找敌人，敌人或朋友有赖于制度基础设施的力量，以及发生规则改变的速度。

重组需要在安全制度的各个方面进行重大的范式转换。根本的范式变化是，安全"最重要也最不重要"。根据当前范例构成的安全制度，应考虑到社会经济发展及其对社会的思考，从多维度、有计划的战略角度实施变革和转型。

每个经济部门的安全化和安全/国防部门每个方面的经济化是需要统一管理的基本范式。如今，传统的基于层次结构的组织及其开展业务的方式已被替代，灵活、模块化、动态的公共生态系统以需求为导向并已完成其数字化转型，这样的公共生态系统对每个人来说都是"浴火凤凰"。（杜鹃翻译）

原文：

Economy, Power and Securiy in the Post-COVID-19 World

Süleyman Şensoy [*]

After the new type coronavirus was identified as "SARS-CoV-2" (Se-

---

* Süleyman Şensoy, Chairman, Turkish Asian Center for Strategic Studies, Turkey.

vere Acute Respiratory Syndrome Coronavirus 2), the global outbreak of the virus was declared as a "pandemic" by the World Health Organization (WHO) and the international arena faced an unexpected crisis.

Especially in the last 12 years, macro and sectoral "strategic transformation" proposals and risk analyses developed by TASAM ingenuity and embodied by numerous projects/programs/reports unfortunately have not been appreciated enough in public, private and civil society in Turkey and the shared countries at the slightest expression. The evolving COVID-19 Pandemic is the first step to confirm these recommendations and analyses. The right-time capture of the power and property model, which is transformed by accelerated traumas, especially the security and defense ecosystem, has become much more difficult with the pandemic.

Global governance; while following the balancing processes with technological, economic, military and political threats, the pandemic faced all actors with a scenario in which they were not ready. Ensuring life security has risen to the top of the world agenda in the international arena, and while markets, international trade and inter-country transportation have come to a halt. Many national infrastructure and economies have been found to be inadequate. This global epidemic is a lesson for the Great Powers, who have left soft areas such as health systems in second place. Unpredictable situations, such as how many waves the outbreak will continue, vaccine studies and possible side effects will occur, require time estimates and scenarios to be kept up-to-date. The absence of economic and political strategy / infrastructure of many actors in the current and future projections of the pandemic is the precursor of the change and transformation imposed by a global crisis.

The concept of "Controlled Governance" seems to be a candidate to be the basic paradigm for every country that does not lose control of its infrastructure. Whatever the name of the next virus or sophisticated crisis, the current pandemic is a global school, but the main thing is; to be able to protect the economic, social and security infrastructure that will apply the lessons learned. As we understand the extraordinary risks of demographic consequences of countries stopping life, it will be better understood that intensive care, intubation and death numbers should be looked at, not the number of cases. Minimized losses are the best option for the bad. Again, food, water and health security has become the top priority and area of cooperation for states and global governance.

The experienced pandemic is a critical milestone for the change of production, consumption, growth and conventional power standards, including security. The reinterpretation of the national and international immune system, scenarios and preparations for strategic transformation has now been the top priority. In this context, "Future Security Ecosystem and its Strategic Transformation", proactively suggested at the highest level by TASAM to many countries along with Turkey long ago, has become a locomotive priority for each country.

It is quite difficult to predict what the next sophisticated crisis area or outbreak will be. As a flare, the current pandemic reveals that; in much of the world threats to security are not likely to arise from the armies of other countries but from a series of problems, such as economic collapse, political oppression, famine, excessive population growth, ethnic divisions, wars, internal conflicts, regional and national conflicts, destruction of nature and the environment, terrorism, organized crime, acts of government violence against its own people, "epidemics", dangerous goods, and smuggling of people, arms and drug trafficking, money laundering, massive financial fraud aimed at destabilizing the market of emerging democracies.

The global financial crisis of 2007 – 2008, "Occupy Wall Street" protests started in the US in 2011, student and activist protests in London, Frankfurt and Paris, "Arab revolts" which exercise influence over and humanitarian crises in sub-Saharan Africa and East Asia; the debates on law and politics, security and freedoms, populism, pluralism and democracy, fault lines related to religious, ethnic, class, racial and minorities, together with the pandemic (mainly including in Western countries) has become much more fragile.

While the effectiveness, inadequacy and changing of international organizations are being discussed, eyes are turned to the economic status of the states as the virus rapidly increases its impact on the whole world. The end of coercion and preferences, which simultaneously bring public, private and household indebtedness to new heights in order to mitigate the effects of the crisis, are not manageable. Moreover, many countries governed by these indicators will not be able to speak of political independence or even maintain stability.

The emergence of such an effective deterrent should be one of the factors that should be questioned in the first place by all states when discussing how beneficial international structures such as WHO, IMF and the EU are for the global system. In the new international order and security regulation, alliances and differences between national and global capacities instead of classical parties will determine the severity and length of the turbulence. In this context, in order to define the new geopolitics, there is an obligation to study formulas that have not been used before. The future of international order and institutions that will be shaped within the framework of "Micro-nationalism" "Integration" and "Unpredictability" depends on a vision of the world supported by "Power and Justice".

The most valuable period of lands was the "Age of Empires". With the "Industrial Revolution", machinery became more valuable. After all, nation-states were born. The "Information Age" we are in today is an international system that promotes micro-nationalism. It would not be an exaggeration to predict that the pandemic can accelerate physical confirmations on this matter. It should also be underlined that "Micro-nationalism" is not about ethnicity (even people who unite around cryptocurrencies can be included within a framework of micro-nationalism) and any organizational difference can be perceived as micro-nationalism.

It is "Critical Thought" and "Merit" that provide the basic regulation for success in the competition of the new era. In fact, the power of the "institutional infrastructure" must be revealed by reinterpreting these parameters, which have been a reference throughout world history, within today's conditions. In addition, at this point in the world's civilization stalemate, the international system, which was constructed after the Second World War-under highly idealistic conditions compared to today-needs to be reinterpreted on the basis of "Power and Justice". Otherwise it would be unlikely to mention a manageable world or country profile. Again, to support this "institutional infrastructure", the area of expertise in managing unpredictability and contrasts-even if it develops by dealing with crises in practice-needs to be developed more consciously and in a fictitious way.

The concept of "Power and Ownership of Power" is changing rapidly, as we have stated for many years. Everything that is conventional; especially the masses of large armies, large crowds, large civil servants and experts, the pandemic will further increase the rate of change of the defense industry capacities, or the institutions that support them (including those producing companies) even more conventional one. It is clear that in a period when information expresses value alone or even outstrips current currencies, a constantly updated search for what the new conventional should be is needed. In this context, the world is entering a period in which the market value of conventional accumulation rapidly melts. This can be a wealth of real estate for people, their vehicles or investment tools and their armies for states. It will be decisive in the new distribution of power to focus on what the new convention is, what its economic counterpart is, and how it should be transformed.

In the business model that will be transformed in the Post-Corona process, to track and deepen the traces of the ecologic breath led by the slowdown in production will ensure that one of the important opportunities arising from the crisis is not wasted. Again, an "expectation management" capacity that will manage the multi-dimensional traumas of the pandemic in social layers will be the key to socio-economic security for public administrations.

For all countries, developing their own infrastructure conventionally for the problems that may arise in the interstate systems and continually improve their economy, military etc. based advances are losing their importance with the pandemic. States with high unemployment rates and economically vulnerable countries are struggling with the threat of collapse of their institutional and systemic infrastructure due to the virus.

It is unknown whether the information and knowledge that was valuable yesterday can maintain its value in the future or even today. In such a turbulent time, it is vital to develop critical strategies in the medium-and long-term plans of the states.

In the global economy, beyond the current corona process, an economic stagnation that will continue in the post-corona period is envisaged. It is considered that the effects of contraction will be long-lasting, with economic contraction occurring at national, regional and global scale. The forecasts are that the global economy will shrink by 4% – 5% this year. It is stated that this level of stagnation and decline in the global economy; will result in stagnation in the assets of international capital and production investments with limited capacity, and in shrinking the capital of foreign subsidiaries.

In this context, it seems that the infrastructures and risk management of the institutions are not sufficient against this negative situation, which has the effect of bringing many more sectors such as manufacturing being in the first place, real estate, commercial and administrative activities; wholesale and retail trade, motor vehicles and logistics; transport, storage and communication; accommodation and food services; arts, shows, entertainment and other services to a standstill.

It is also possible that the current shrinkage and recession make a war-free global correction and could give a breath to the resource crisis in the "debt-money-debt" spiral. But in this case, the relative welfare sharing in the distribution of debt and capital will continue to deteriorate unbelievably for humanity.

According to recent evaluations by economists, the global economy is estimated to take a knock around 5. 5 trillion dollars due to the pandemic. The losses in the derivative markets have reaching tens of trillion dollars and the number of people at risk of loss of employment has approaching 1 billion. It is estimated that the cost of the pandemic to the economies of developed countries will be above the levels of the 1929, 2008 – 2009 and 1975 recessions experienced in the past periods. It is also among the predictions that the return to economic levels before Corona will occur only in 2023.

The global business model, distribution of power and property, security and defense; will be transformed by the core sectors "Robotics" "Biotechnology" "Artificial Intelligence" "Nanotechnology" "Space" and "Strategic Services" that have been confirmed once again with the pandemic. Again, the crises have made visible the definitions of the concepts of "security" and "power" in the new strategic environment that has been persistently expressed for the past 15 years. This situation requires the institutions and their stakeholders operating in the areas of defence, security, diplomacy and socio-economy to re-organize by reinterpreting these new conventional concepts. In this context, it is the most important awareness for countries to see that there is no need to look for enemies inside and out, that the enemy or friend is in the power of institutional infrastructure and at the speed of producing regulation change.

Re-organization requires an important paradigm shift in all aspects of security institutions. The fundamental paradigm change is that security is "everything and nothing. " Security institutions structured according to the current paradigm; It should implement change and transformation from a multi-dimensional and planned strategic perspective, taking into account socio-economic developments and their reflections on society.

The securitization of each economic sector and the economization of each dimension of the security/defense sector are the basic paradigms that need to be managed together. Now, instead of traditional hierarchy-based organizations and the way they do business, what and how the public ecosystem that is flexible, modular, dynamic, fluid, needs-oriented and has completed its digital transformation is a phoenix for everyone.

希望之路

王琇德（Soo Deok Wang）*

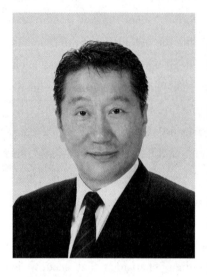

新冠肺炎疫情为全人类带来了前所未有的挑战。大多数人，甚至包括那些百岁以上的老人都从未经历过如此大规模的疫情。许多人都感到困惑，无法确定是什么原因加剧了病毒的传播。这次疫情证明，人类从来都不是不可战胜的，甚至在大自然的考验面前不堪一击。全世界各国意识到这次疫情已发展成为全球范围的考验。随着疫情的蔓延，中国国家主席习近平作出重要讲话，强调人类命运共同体理念。现在看来，这一理念正变得比以往任何时候都更清楚、重要。在这次疫情中，自私自利的个人主义失去了施展的空间，而且人们也清楚地意识到在这危机时刻，任何形式的个人主义都不应该存在。在面对威胁全人类生存的巨大挑战时，闭关锁国和人民对立等概念一下子变得过时老旧，我们也终于理解了大团结的真正含义。

在这场与新型冠状病毒的战斗中，不同的国家和地区采取了不同的应对策略。同时，每个国家也展现了不同程度的领导和调动能力。由于各国的领导体制基础不同，无法评论好坏，但我们仍能看出哪些

---

* 王琇德，韩国中华总商会常务副会长兼事务处长、秘书长。

国家的领导体制效率较高。一些国家的领导体制在疫情发生前显得稳固且强大，但在疫情面前被证明是低效无能的。相反，一些平日里不显山不露水的国家却在此次疫情中迸发出强大的领导力，并为全人类指明了一条生存和发展之路。自诞生之日起，马克思主义便一直与其他各种意识形态相竞争。而在应对疫情方面，马克思主义被证实是一种最有效的意识形态，中国的应对方式也为全世界提供着宝贵经验。此外，虽然没有明说，但我们能感觉到全世界的人们都在效仿和学习中国的做法。

中国对抗新型冠状病毒的战争已接近尾声，疫情目前已得到基本控制，这为恢复国内经济生产活动奠定了基础。全球对抗新型冠状病毒的战争终将获胜，全球的经济也将逐步恢复。疫情之后，全球将如何迈向更美好的未来、哪个国家会成为新的领头羊？全球经济的规则和秩序将会重新洗牌。我认为，这些经济规则在制定的过程中需要各方仔细审核、广泛磋商。但是，关于哪个国家应该在疫情结束后引领全球发展，每个人心里都有一杆秤。无端的指责无法改变这一事实。
（董方源翻译）

原文：

A Road to Hope

Soo Deok Wang [*]

The COVID-19 Pandemic presented an unprecedented challenge to the human race. Most of the people, even those over the age of one hundred,

---

* Soo Deok Wang, Vice President, Overseas Chinese Chambers of Commerce in Korea.

have never experienced anything like the pandemic. Many are confounded and unsure of what exacerbated the havoc. The pandemic made it clear that the human race is never invincible and is vulnerable to the test of nature. The world realized that the pandemic is a test for the entire world. As the test carries out, president Xi's remark that we are living under the Community with a Shared Future for Mankind is becoming more clear than ever. In the outbreak, there is now no room for selfish individualism, and it is clear that there should not be any room. Facing the challenge that threatens the existence of us all, the concept of separate nation and people became obsolete; we finally came to understand what the Great Unity is.

Under the joint fight against the virus, different countries and regions adopted different strategies against the virus. Each country exhibited different leadership. Though each leadership has its own basis and we cannot evaluate which is better, we can certainly see which leadership is of effectiveness. Leadership which seemed powerful before proved ineffective in front of the new virus, and on the contrary, what we did not see during the normal days brought about a strong leadership effect and showed to the human race a road for survival and development. Marxism has been competing with other ideologies since its birth, but in terms of coping with the pandemic, Marxism is proven to be one of the most effective; China's way is leading the world. In addition, though not explicitly expressed, the people throughout the world are following and learning China's way.

The fight against the virus is heading towards the end in China. The outbreak is coming under control, and the country has laid the foundation to resume its economic activity. Ultimately, the global fight against the virus will be over, and the global economy will also recover. Afterwards, there will be new rules for the global economy concerning how the world should build towards a better future and which country should lead the way in the post-pandemic age. The rules, in my view, will require careful scrutiny and much conference. However, in everyone's mind there is a clear answer on which country should lead the post-pandemic age. Unfounded blame cannot change this fact.

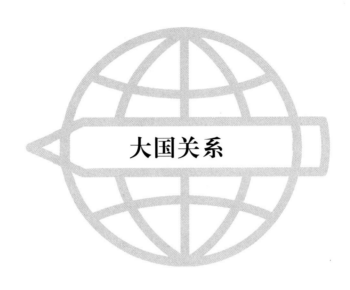

大国关系

复杂时代的大国关系

马凯硕（Kishore Mahbubani）*

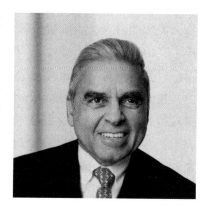

　　犹如驶入复杂海域的船只，大国关系正进入变幻莫测的时期。因为我们的世界秩序正在重新洗牌。很多世界大国尚不知如何面对这些大规模的转型。或许可以制定一个简单的框架，即一个多极、多文明和多边的框架来及时阐释世界将如何作出改变。

　　在这个变幻莫测的时期，美中两国之间正在进行一场至关重要的地缘政治博弈。正如我在《中国赢了吗》一书中所述，这场地缘政治博弈貌似不可避免，但实际上又可避免。许多中国人感到困惑的是，美国为何选在世界面临诸多危机之际发起这场斗争。因此，本文将试图解释驱使美国进入地缘政治博弈的深层心理动机。在了解了地缘政治、文明转型和多边秩序所发生的重大变化之后，才能更好地理解这些变化。

　　在地缘政治领域，美国正在经历一次严重的心理创伤，因为它面临一个拐点，即美苏冷战（1947—1991年）之后的美国单极时代即将结束。1950年前后，美国在全球GNP中的份额约为50%。这是一个惊人的数字，因为美国只有世界人口的5%。因此，《生活杂志》的创办人和所有者亨利·卢斯（Henry Luce）理所当然地将之称为

"美国世纪"。

显然，这个"美国世纪"即将结束。因为就真实购买力（PPP）而言，美国现在是世界第二大经济体（中国是第一大经济体）。这个变化速度让人震撼。1980 年，美国的真实购买力是中国的十倍；到 2014 年，差距已经变小。按名义市场计算，美国 20.5 万亿美元的国内生产总值（GDP）仍远大于中国的 13.6 万亿美元。既然美国的 GDP 仍然大得多，美国应该感到强大和自信。不幸的是，美国人民不仅没有从最近的经济增长中获益，反而有 50% 的美国底层民众的平均收入在 30 年中呈下降趋势。正如普林斯顿大学的两位经济学家所言，美国的白人工人阶级中形成了一片"绝望的海洋"，这产生了民粹主义的政治冲动，导致了 2016 年唐纳德·特朗普总统的当选。可以说，美国不是一个让人有幸福感的国度。

相比之下，在过去的五十年里，中国有 50% 的人民群众的生活水平获得有史以来最大的提高。斯坦福大学心理学家范让（Jean Fan）表示，"与美国的经济停滞形成鲜明对比的是，中国的文化、自我认知和士气正在发生飞速转变——主要是为了更好的发展"①。与此同时，其他亚洲国家也发展良好。就真实购买力而言，世界四大经济体是中国、美国、印度和日本。可以说，20 世纪是"美国世纪"，而 21 世纪将成为"亚洲世纪"。

为了应对这种大规模的权力转移，美国采取的一个明智策略是，集中精力重振国内"精神活力"。事实上，美国最聪明的战略思想家之一乔治·凯南（George Kennan）在 1949 年就有先见之明地告诉他的美国同胞，与苏联冷战的结果将取决于美国是否能保持相关领域的领导者地位。可悲的是，在 2020 年，美国领导人无视他的明智建议。更可悲的是，美国最亲密的朋友和盟友，包括其欧洲伙伴以及澳大利亚、加拿大和新西兰，也没有建议美国专注于国内发展，而不是与中国进行不必要的地缘政治博弈。为什么美国的西方伙伴和盟友没有提出如此明智的建议？

①　Kishore Mahbubani, *Has China Won?: The Chinese Challenge to American Primacy*, New York: Public Affairs, 2020, p. 12.

188

答案来自世界发展进程中的第二次重大转折：我们正在从19世纪和20世纪西方文明主导的单一文明世界，转向一个由中国文明、印度文明，日本和西方文明共同组成的多元文明世界。在西方主宰世界历史的时代，包括欧洲和澳大利亚在内的所有西方社会都在世界秩序中享有特权地位。他们对世界其他地区有一种文化优越感。而现在西方必须面对其他同样自信的文明。澳大利亚必须做出特别艰难的心理转变，学会给予亚洲文化更多的尊重。

中国不是唯一受到西方文化挑战的亚洲国家。令人惊讶的是，印度也有类似遭遇。当欧盟（EU）与印度谈判自由贸易协定时，欧盟试图将人权标准强加于印度。时任外交国务部部长的沙希·塔鲁尔（Shashi Tharoor）就此回应道："印度人对被训话过敏，欧印伙伴关系的一大失误是欧洲倾向于向印度训话……"[1]

尽管存在这些困难，但在一个多文明的世界里，西方仍可以毫不费力地接近印度。西方并不惧怕印度。然而，正如我在《中国赢了吗》一书中所言，"西方精神的潜意识中深藏着对'黄祸论'朦胧又真实的恐惧"[2]。这种对"黄祸论"的恐惧解释了为何欧盟（或许还有澳大利亚）在新的多极地缘政治环境中没有表现出理性的地缘政治行为。

欧盟对重要的地缘政治挑战问题做出理性而冷静的分析。该分析表明，其主要挑战将来自非洲。1950年，欧盟的总人口（3.79亿）几乎是非洲（2.29亿）的两倍。现在，非洲人口（2015年为12亿）是欧盟国家的两倍（2018年为5.13亿）。到2100年，非洲人口（45亿）预计将是欧洲（4.93亿）的近10倍。鉴于地理临近，非洲人口将很容易流入欧洲。我们已经看到，一波又一波的移民潮在欧洲引发了民粹主义运动，扭曲了欧洲社会的中间派自由主义倾向。因此，与其他伙伴合作，促进非洲的长期经济发展，符合欧盟长期的利益。最好的合作伙伴是中国，因为中国正在成为非洲

---

[1] Kishore Mahbubani, *Has China Won？*：*The Chinese Challenge to American Primacy*, New York：Public Affairs, 2020, p. 277.

[2] Kishore Mahbubani, *Has China Won？*：*The Chinese Challenge to American Primacy*, New York：Public Affairs, 2020, p. 258.

最大的新投资者。然而，出于文化原因，在美中地缘政治的博弈中，尽管欧洲自身的地缘政治利益指向了与中国的合作，但欧洲却倾向于支持美国。

或许多文明世界给西方国家带来了不适。但在我们这个需要彼此依存、共同应对全球挑战（如新冠肺炎疫情和全球变暖）的小星球上，对多边主义的需求正日益增长。这可能导致一种新的全球秩序，这个秩序有助于抑制美中之间的斗争。当今，法国总统马克龙是多边主义的最权威发言人。他说："全球化和多边主义产生了不可低估的积极影响：它们使地球上数亿居民摆脱了贫困，结束了分裂世界的意识形态冲突，他们开创了一个空前繁荣和自由的时代，并和平地扩大了全球贸易，这是近几十年来都存在的事实。"当前全球正遭受新型冠状病毒的威胁、世界经济衰退，大多数欧洲国家和其他国家都对特朗普政府决定撤回对世界卫生组织（WHO）的资助感到震惊。

这为中国创造了最好的地缘政治机遇，因为中国正试图应对美国发起的这场艰难的地缘政治之战。这场地缘政治博弈中，让中国特别难以应对的是，美国在发动地缘政治博弈时，没有率先制定出全面且长期的战略，这是基辛格在一对一午餐会上向我提供的见解。由于缺乏相关战略，美国成为一个非常不可捉摸，甚至非理性的地缘政治竞争对手。新冠肺炎疫情的暴发凸显了这种不合理性。地缘政治的经典规则之一是，敌人的敌人是我的朋友。由于新冠肺炎疫情是美国的主要敌人（其杀害的美国人比两次世界大战中丧生的美国人还多），美国的理性反应应该是与中国合作对付新冠肺炎疫情。可是，特朗普政府却做了相反的事情。

更糟糕的是，随着新冠肺炎疫情在美国的蔓延情况加重，特朗普政府加剧了与中国的地缘政治斗争。从理论上说，特朗普政府会因没有与中国合作对付共同敌人而受到反对党民主党的批评。但恰恰相反，民主党人支持特朗普。这清楚地证明，在美国的政治体制中，两党已经形成了一种强烈的共识，即美国已经到了与中国抗衡的时候了。因此，即使乔·拜登在2020年11月的选举中击败唐纳德·特朗普，美中地缘政治之战也不会停歇，尽管乔·拜登在公开场合会对中国更加彬彬有礼。不过，如果拜登当选，也会对中国产生不利因素，因为在拜登执政后，西方国家将再次向美国靠拢。

如果西方在美中地缘政治角逐中与中国势均力敌（出于文明团结，而非合理的地缘政治的考虑），中国将不会孤军奋战。西方占世界人口的12%，甚至比中国的人口还要少。世界其他地区仍有超过50亿人口。这些地区的大多数国家都希望专注于本国的社会和经济发展，而不被地缘政治斗争分散注意。他们赞成加强全球多边机构的作用。

在多极化、多文明的世界秩序中，中国应对美中地缘政治博弈的最佳选择是努力构建全球多边机构。事实上，2017年1月习近平主席在达沃斯和日内瓦发表演讲时对此表示赞成。他说："要坚持多边主义，维护多边体制权威性和有效性。要践行承诺、遵守规则，不能按照自己的意愿取舍或选择。"他还说："我们要下大气力发展全球互联互通，让世界各国实现联动增长，走向共同繁荣。我们要坚定不移发展全球自由贸易和投资，在开放中推动贸易和投资自由化便利化，旗帜鲜明反对保护主义。"

随着时间的推移，更强大的全球多边秩序将有力遏制1990—2020年单极时代美国政策制定中占了上风的单边主义行为。更重要的是，这个更强大的全球多边秩序实际上也将有利于美国人民的利益。2003年，美国前总统比尔·克林顿明智地建议美国同胞，美国应努力创造"一个有规则、有伙伴关系和行为习惯的世界，当我们不再是世界上军事、政治和经济超级大国时，我们愿意生活在这个世界上"。在未来几十年，中美两国之间的这场至关重要的地缘政治博弈几乎不可避免，但正如我在《中国赢了吗》一书中所言，这也为中国创造了新的地缘政治机会，特别是在多边领域，可能会缓慢而稳定地逐步化解这场大规模的地缘政治较量。（王晶翻译）

原文：

Major Country Relations in an Era of Complexity

Kishore Mahbubani *

Humanity is sailing into a sea of complexity. Why? Because we are experiencing massive changes across multiple dimensions in our world order. This explains also the sense of bewilderment among the major countries of the world on how to manage these massive transitions. Yet, it is also possible to work out a simple framework to understand how our world is becoming transformed. It is becoming, simultaneous, multi-polar, multi-civilizational and multilateral.

In the middle of this sea of complexity, a major geopolitical contest has broken out between the US and China. As I documented in my book, *Has China Won?* This geopolitical contest is both inevitable and avoidable. Many Chinese are puzzled that the US decided to launch this contest at a time when our world is facing many pressing common challenges. This essay will therefore try to explain some of the deep psychological impulses driving the US into this contest. They can best be understood after we have understood the major changes taking place in geopolitics, civilizational transformations and the multilateral orders.

In the field of geopolitics, the US is experiencing a major psychological

* Kishore Mahbubani, a Distinguished Fellow at the Asia Research Institute, National University of Singapore, is the author of *Has China Won?*: *The Chinese Challenge to American Primacy* (Public Affairs, 2020) .

trauma as its establishment comes to grips with the new reality that the uni-polar era, which succeeded the bipolar era of the Cold War from 1947 to 1991, is coming to an end. The American share of the Global SNP was al-most 50% around 1950. This was an astonishing share by America, which had only 5% of the world's population. As a result, Henry Luce, the found-er and owner of *Life* magazine could justifiably call it the American Century.

This American Century is clearly coming to an end. Indeed in purcha-sing power parity (PPP) terms, the US has become the number two econo-my in the world. It's quite shocking how fast this has happened. In 1980, the American economy was ten times larger than China in PPP terms. By 2014, it had become smaller. In nominal market terms, the US GDP is still much bigger than China, US \$ 20. 5 trillion versus US \$ 13. 6 trillion. Since the American GDP is still much bigger, the US should feel strong and self-confi-dent. Sadly, the American people haven't benefitted from recent American e-conomic growth. Indeed, the average income of the bottom fifty percent has gone down over a thirty-year period, creating, as two Princeton University e-conomists have described, a "sea of despair" among the white working clas-ses in America, which in turn has generated the populist political impulses that have led to the election of President Donald Trump in 2016. America is not a happy country.

By contrast, over the past fifty years, the bottom fifty percent in China have probably experienced the greatest improvement in their standard of liv-ing that the Chinese people have experienced in four thousand years. Jean Fan, a Stanford University Psychologist, says "In contrast to America's stagnation, China's culture, self-concept and morale are being transformed at a rapid pace-mostly for the better."[1] At the same time, other Asian soci-eties are doing well. In PPP terms, the four largest economies of the world are China, the US, India and Japan. The American century of the 20th cen-tury will become the "Asian century" of the 21st century.

① Kishore Mahbubani, *Has China Won?*: *The Chinese Challenge to American Primacy*, New York: Public Affairs, 2020, p. 12.

A wise American strategy in response to this massive shift of power would be to focus on revitalizing its domestic "spiritual vitality". Indeed, one of America's wisest strategic thinkers, George Kennan, had presciently advised his fellow Americans in 1949 that the outcome of the Cold War with the Soviet Union would depend on America preserving its lead in this area. Sadly, in 2020, America's leaders are ignoring his wise advice. Even more sadly, America's closest friends and allies including its European partners and Australia, Canada and New Zealand, are also not advising America to focus on its domestic development, not its unnecessary geopolitical contest with China. Why aren't America's Western partners and allies providing such wise advice?

The answer is given by the second big shift happening in the world: we are moving away from the mono-civilizational world of the 19th and 20th centuries, dominated by one successful civilization, the Western Civilization, towards a world where we are seeing many successful civilizations, including Chinese, Indian, Japanese and Western civilizations. In the era of Western domination of world history, all Western societies, including Europe and Australia, enjoyed privileged positions in the world order. They felt a sense of cultural superiority vis-a-vis the rest of the world. Now the West has to deal with other equally self-confident civilizations. Australia has to make a particularly difficult psychological transition as it has to learn to treat its Asian neighbours with greater cultural respect.

China is not the only Asian country to receive cultural condescension from the West. Surprisingly, India has received similar treatment. When the European Union (EU) was negotiating a free-trade agreement with India, the EU tried to impose human rights standards on India. The then Minister of State for External Affairs Shashi Tharoor wrote in response, "Indians have an allergy to being lectured to, and one of the great failings in the EU-India partnership has been the tendency of Europe to preach to India…"[1].

---

[1] Kishore Mahbubani, *Has China Won?: The Chinese Challenge to American Primacy*, New York: Public Affairs, 2020, p. 277.

Despite these difficulties, the West will have no problem getting close to India in a multi-civilizational world. The West doesn't fear India. However, as I documented in *Has China Won?* "there has been buried deep in the unconsciousness of the western psyche an inchoate but real fear of the 'yellow peril'." [1] This fear of the "yellow peril" explains why the European Union (and perhaps Australia) are not behaving as rational geopolitical actor in our new multi-polar geopolitical environment.

A rational and dispassionate analysis of the EU's major geopolitical challenges will show that its main challenge will come from Africa. In 1950, the EU's combined population (379 million) was nearly double that of Africa's (229 million). Today, Africa's population (1.2 billion in 2015) is double that of the EU countries (513 million in 2018). By 2100, Africa's population is projected to be almost ten times larger at 4.5 billion versus 493 million. Given the geographical proximity, Africa's population will spill over into Europe easily. We have already seen how small waves of migrants have sparked populist movements in Europe, distorting the centrist liberal tendencies of European societies. It is therefore in EU's rational long-term interest to work with other partners to foster the long-term economic development of Africa. The best partner would be China, since China is emerging as the largest new investor in Africa. Yet, for cultural reasons, Europe is leaning towards the US in the US-China geopolitical contest, even though its own geopolitical interests point in the direction of working with China also.

Yet, if the multicivilizational world is creating discomfort for the Western countries, the growing demand for multilateralism in our small interdependent planet, facing many common global challenges (like COVID-19 and global warming), could result in a new global order that could help to restrain US-China rivalry. The most eloquent spokesperson for multilateralism today is President Macron of France. He has said, "Globalization and multilateralism have had positive effects that should not be underestimated: they

---

① Kishore Mahbubani, *Has China Won?: The Chinese Challenge to American Primacy*, New York: Public Affairs, 2020, p. 258.

enabled hundreds of millions of the planet's inhabitants to escape poverty, they brought an end to an ideological conflict that divided the world, and they ushered in an unprecedented era of prosperity and freedom and a peaceful expansion of global trade, which is the reality of recent decades. " Most European countries, together with the rest of the world, were shocked by the decision of the Trump Administration to withdraw funding of the World Health Organisation (WHO) when the world was threatened by COVID-19.

This creates the best geopolitical opportunity for China as it tries to manage the difficult geopolitical contest that the US has launched against it. What makes this geopolitical contest particularly difficult for China to handle is that the US has launched the geopolitical contest without first working out a comprehensive long-term strategy, an insight provided to me by Henry Kissinger at a one-to-one lunch. This lack of a strategy makes the US a very unpredictable, even irrational, geopolitical competitor. The irrationality was shown when COVID-19 broke out. One of the oldest rules of geopolitics is that the enemy of my enemy is my friend. Since COVID-19 is a major enemy of the US (killing more Americans than in the two world wars that the US fought), the rational response of the US should have been to work with China against COVID-19. Instead, the Trump Administration did the opposite.

Worse still, the Trump Administration has stepped up the geopolitical contest with China as COVID-19 kept gaining momentum in the US. In theory, this should have led to the opposing party, the Democrats, to criticize the Trump Administration for not cooperating with China against a common enemy. Instead, the opposite happened. The Democrats supported Trump. This provides clear proof that a strong bipartisan consensus has developed in the American body politic that the time had come for the US to stand up to China. Hence, even if Joe Biden defeats Donald Trump in the election in November 2020, there will be no respite in the US-China geopolitical contest, although Joe Biden will be more publicly courteous towards China. However, there will also be a downside for China if Biden is elected. The

Western countries will move closer again to the US in a Biden Administration.

If the West closes ranks against China in the US-China geopolitical contest (out of civilizational solidarity, not sound geopolitical calculations), China will not be alone. The West represents 12% of the world's population, which is even smaller than China's population. That still leaves over 5 billion people in the rest of the world. Most of the remaining countries of the world want to focus on their internal social and economic development and not get distracted by geopolitical contests. They are also in favour of strengthening global multilateral institutions.

China's best option in managing the US-China geopolitical contest in a multi-polar and multi-civilizational world order is to work towards strengthening global multilateral institutions. Indeed, President Xi Jinping spoke out in favour of this when he skope in Davos and Geneva in January 2017. He said, "We should adhere to multilateralism to uphold the authority and efficacy of multilateral institutions. We should honor promises and abide by rules. One should not select or bend rules as he sees fit. " He has also said, "We must redouble efforts to develop global connectivity to enable all countries to achieve inter-connected growth and share prosperity. We must remain committed to developing global free trade and investment, promote trade and investment liberalization and facilitation through opening-up and say no to protectionism. "

Over time, a stronger global multilateral order will provide the best checks to the unilateral impulses that have prevailed in American policymaking in the unipolar era of 1991 – 2020. Even more importantly, a stronger global multilateral order will actually work in favour of the interests of the American people also. In 2003, former President Bill Clinton wisely advised his fellow Americans that the US should work towards creating "a world with rules and partnerships and habits of behavior that we would like to live in when we're no longer the military, political and economic superpower in the world. " Hence, even though a major geopolitical contest between the US and China is virtually unstoppable in the coming decades, as I documented in *Has China Won?* It can also create new geopolitical opportunities for China, especially in the multilateral arena, which could lead slowly and steadily towards a gradual defusing of this massive geopolitical contest.

疫情后中美关系将进入
一个更困难时期

当前，百年未有的大疫情仍在全球肆虐。人们的普遍看法是，疫情之后，世界将变得与以往大不相同。实际上，在世界正在发生的变化中，最大因变量是美国，以及由此带来的中美关系的变化。在疫情期间，由于特朗普政府不断对中国进行指责和发难，本应携手抗击疫情的中国和美国之间非但没能进行有效的合作，反而出现了关系的急剧下滑。这预示着在走出疫情之后，中美关系将进入一个更加困难的时期。

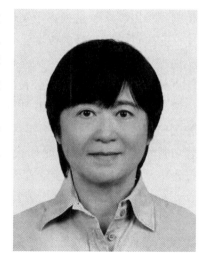

美国已认定中国为战略竞争对手

中美关系的重大转折发生在特朗普总统当政之后。美国对中国的基本判断发生了深刻变化。这一变化来自两条主线，一个是战略方面的，另一个是经贸方面的。

　＊　周琪，同济大学全球治理与发展研究院院长，中国社会科学院美国研究所研究员。

从战略方面来看，与中美关系有关的各项条件都在恶化。在特朗普政府 2017 年 12 月发布的《美国国家安全战略报告》和 2018 年 1 月发布的《美国国防战略报告》中，中国被认定为"修正主义的竞争者"，"挑战美国的实力、影响和利益，试图侵蚀美国的安全和繁荣"。"随着中国继续扩大其经济和军事优势，并通过一个全国性的长期战略扩大其权力，其将继续推行军事现代化计划，旨在在近期寻求印太地区的区域霸权，在将来驱逐美国，实现全球领先。"

两年多后，特朗普政府对中国的这一看法再次被确认。2020 年 5 月 20 日白宫发布的《美国对中华人民共和国的战略方针》声称：中共正在利用自由和开放的国际秩序，以有利于它的方式重塑国际体系和改变国际秩序，并"越来越多地使用经济、政治和军事力量强迫民族国家予以默认，这损害了美国至关重要的利益"。

美国对中国战略的改变，是出于对中美实力和影响力对比变化的深切担忧。美国战略界今天终于不再讳言美国相对实力的下降了。曾任克林顿政府助理国防部部长的著名国际关系学家格雷厄姆·艾利森注意到，在 21 世纪的前 20 年里发生了国家权力格局的戏剧性变化，美国国内生产总值从 1991 年占全球的 1/4 下降到今天仅占 1/7；美国著名智库战略与国际问题研究中心在最近发表的《创新优势战略》报告中承认，"美国的全球首要地位正在下降，而且不太可能回归"。

在对中国的政策上，美国国会中的两党议员表现出惊人的一致。此外，一个引人注目的动向是，2020 年 5 月 7 日，美国众议院共和党领袖麦卡锡宣布将在众议院成立一个共和党的"中国特别工作小组"，其中包括国家安全、科技、经济与能源、竞争力和意识形态竞争五个支柱小组，它们将就中国构成的威胁提出各自的政策建议。

美国民众对中国的看法也在发生变化。2020 年 4 月 21 日，皮尤研究中心发表的民调报告显示，66% 的美国民众对华持负面看法，只有 26% 的美国民众持正面看法，这是 2005 年开始这项调查以来的最高纪录。90% 的美国民众将中国视为"威胁"，其中 62% 的人认为中国是"主要威胁"，这一结果比 2018 年上升了 14 个百分点。

美国挑起的对中国的贸易摩擦不会停止

从经贸方面来看，美国把自身经济出现的所有问题都归咎于中国。2017 年 3 月，即特朗普总统上任后仅 2 个月，美国政府就发布了《总统 2017 年贸易政策日程》，声称自 2000 年，即中国加入 WTO 前一年以来，美国的各项经济指标就在持续恶化：GDP 增长放缓、就业增长缓慢、制造业就业人数大幅度减少、贸易逆差加大。该文件由此得出一个结论：目前的全球贸易体系对中国是有利的，但对美国不利。美国不应再为了获得地缘政治优势而对其在全球市场中遇到的不公平贸易做法视而不见，要"使美国再度伟大"，就必须消除中国所造成的贸易"不公平"。为此，特朗普政府从 2018 年 3 月起，开始对中国输美商品加征关税，而中国则被迫开始同美国进行漫长而艰难的贸易谈判。

疫情暴发之后，由于疫情在一段时期阻断了产业供应链，对于一些发达国家来说，从中国撤资或将生产线转移到中国之外的必要性更具有了说服力。一些国家已经采取了这样的措施：美国政府以优惠政策要求本国企业迁回国内；日本政府建议企业考虑从中国迁走部分工厂，以降低供应链过于单一的风险；欧盟官员在谈论"战略自主权"，并准备建立一项基金来购买公司的股份。国内外许多经济学家都已对此类举动做出评论指出，对美国而言，重建传统工业需要付出巨大代价；美国劳动力成本过高；在机械化和自动化的条件下，即使恢复传统工业也创造不了多少就业岗位；把产业链移出中国，会增添在其他国家重建的成本，可能还会面临较差的投资环境；最重要的是可能会丧失广大的中国市场，等等。由于这些原因，全面的经济脱钩很难实现，但中国对美及其盟友贸易的困难和波动不可避免。

科技脱钩显露端倪

应当看到，特朗普领导下的美国发生这样的转变并非仅由其个人因素所致。研究表明，在过去几十年的快速全球化过程中，最大的受益者是发展中国家的中上阶层和发达国家的高收入群体,而最大的受损者是发达国家的中低收入群体。特朗普以"美国优先"的政策来迎击全球化,激烈地攻击自由贸易和外来移民,他的当选对于那些自认为深受自由贸易之害的美国中下层白人来说是一场胜利,他们也是自由贸易最激烈的反对者和特朗普逆全球化政策坚定的支持者。特朗普的逆全球化行动也不是孤立现象,英国脱欧和欧洲各国极右势力的兴起,都证明深度的全球化反而会激发民粹主义情绪。由于反全球化,美国需要与中国合作的领域就变得愈发狭窄。

国际上不少学者已经指出,在新冠肺炎疫情大流行之前,全球化已经达到了其最大限度。这次疫情促使许多西方国家采取措施抑制全球化。《经济学家》杂志甚至悲哀地宣告,"向全球化的最伟大时代告别"。尽管逆全球化极有可能出现,但有理由认为,受到影响的只是全球化的程度。换言之,全球化仍然是一个大趋势,但其程度可能因一些发达国家逆全球化的措施而有所降低。

尽管中美经济的全面脱钩目前看来不大可能,但科技脱钩的问题却日益凸显出来。美国和其他西方国家现在担心的不仅是其企业和产品的国际竞争力,而更担心的是能否确保国家安全。如今,科技领域里的竞争已被视为战略竞争,对于美国来说还是一场争夺世界领导权的竞争。为此,美国试图采取一切措施来减缓中国科技的发展,包括对外国投资美国核心技术进行更严格的筛选,严密审查中国的学术交流,针对性地增加关税以降低中国在关键领域的竞争力,并在反情报行动中投入更多的资源,以及最近禁止美国公司对中国人工智能产业出口关键产品,以对中国进行科技封锁。不仅如此,美国还要求其他盟友配合其行动。从现有美国和欧洲的政策趋向来看,疫情之后这些措施力度很可能会加大。

国际上更多的人担心,中美之间日益激烈的技术竞争可能导致技术领域的分离,最后导致欧洲、北美、南美和澳大利亚主要采用美国的技术和标准,亚洲、非洲和中东则采用中国的技术和标准,而美国与中国之间在5G标准方面的全球竞争可能是这种脱钩的早期迹象。如果中美贸易紧张局势加剧,美国竭力限制中国的市场,将可能导致形成两个不可兼容的5G生态系统:一个系统由美国领导,并由硅谷开发的技术支持，将主要在竞争激烈的发达国家市场开展业务；而另一个系统由中国领导，并由其强大的数字平台公司提供支持，市场主要集中在发展中国家。从美国目前采取的政策力度来看，这样的结果不是不可想象。

鉴于上述情况，我们必须为疫情之后中美关系将进入一个更困难时期做好应对准备。由于美国国内现存的社会、经济问题，除非美国真正尝到苦果，即其政策后果最终证明事与愿违，其政策不会做出调整，把中国视为头号竞争对手的国家安全战略还会继续下去，一定程度的经济脱钩和最大可能的科技脱钩都是可能出现的。

译文：

China-US Relations in a More Difficult Situation After the Pandemic

Zhou Qi[*]

At present, a pandemic unseen in a hundred years is still rampant across the world. It is widely believed that the world will be very different after the coronavirus. In fact, of the changes taking place in the world, the biggest dependent variable is the US and the resulting changes in China-US relations. As the Trump administration keeps shifting the blame onto China, the two major countries, which should have joined hands in fighting COVID-19, have failed to cooperate effectively, leading to the sharp deterioration of

---

* Zhou Qi, Director, Institute of Global Governance and Development, Tongji University & Researcher, Senior Research Fellow, Institute of American Studies, CASS.

their relations. This indicates that after the coronavirus, China-US relations will get into a more difficult situation.

The US has Identified China as a Strategic Rival

A major turning point in China-US relations came when Donald Trump took office. The US has profoundly changed its basic judgment on China. This change has both strategic and economic causes.

From a strategic point of view, all conditions related to China-US relations are deteriorating. In the National Security Strategy of the United States of America released by the Trump administration in December 2017 and the National Defense Strategy of the United States of America released in January 2018, China is classified as a "revisionist power" that "challenges American power, influence, and interests, attempting to erode American security and prosperity." "As China continues its economic and military ascendance, asserting power through an all-of-nation long-term strategy, it will continue to pursue a military modernization program that seeks Indo-Pacific regional hegemony in the near-term and displacement of the United States to achieve global preeminence in the future."

A bit more than two years later, the Trump administration's view of China was re-confirmed. On May 20, 2020, the White House issued the United States Strategic Approach to the People's Republic of China, claiming that "the CCP has chosen instead to exploit the free and open rules-based order and attempt to reshape the international system in its favor and the CCP's expanding use of economic, political, and military power to compel acquiescence from nation states harms vital American interests."

The change of American strategy towards China is out of the deep concern about the change of strength and influence between China and the United States. Today, the American strategic circle makes no attempt to conceal the fact that the relative power of the US has declined. Graham Allison, a famous expert on international relations who served as Assistant Secretary of

Defense of the Clinton administration, has noticed the dramatic changes in the state power structure in the first 20 years of the 21st century: the US share of global GDP has fallen from one-quarter in 1991 to one-seventh today. The Center for Strategic and International Studies (CSIS), a famous think tank in the US, admitted in the recently published Innovation Superiority Strategy that "US global primacy is declining and unlikely to return. "

Members of the two parties in the US Congress are astonishingly unanimous in the policy toward China. In addition, a striking move is that on May 7, 2020, House Republican Leader Kevin McCarthy announced the formation of a Republican "China Task Force" in the House, which consists of five pillars: national security, science and technology, economics and energy, competitiveness, and ideological competition. They will put forward policy recommendations on the threat posed by China.

US views of China are also changing. According to the poll report released by the Pew Research Center on April 21, 2020, "roughly two-thirds of Americans now have a negative opinion of China, the highest percentage recorded since Pew Research Center began asking the question in 2005. Only 26% report a favorable attitude. About nine-in-ten U. S. adults see China's power and influence as a threat—including 62% who say it is a major threat. The share perceiving China as a major threat has increased 14 percentage points since 2018. "

The US Trade Friction With China Will Not Stop

In economic and trade terms, the US has put the blame for all its economic problems on China. In March 2017, just two months after President Trump assumed office, the US government issued the President's 2017 Trade Policy Agenda, claiming that since 2000, "the last full year before China joined the WTO", the US has witnessed the constant deterioration of its economic indicators: "slowed GDP growth, weak employment growth, a sharp net loss of manufacturing employment", and "a rising trade deficit" . The document concludes that "the current global trading system has been great for China, it has not generated the same results for the United States." The US should no longer, "for putative geopolitical advantage, turn a blind eye to unfair trade practices". To "Make America Great Again", it must eliminate the "unfair" trade caused by China. To this end, the Trump administration began to impose tariffs on Chinese imports from March 2018, while Beijing was forced to start long and difficult trade negotiations with Washington.

As the coronavirus outbreak delayed the industrial supply chain for a period of time, some developed countries have seen a more convincing necessity of withdrawing capital from China or moving production out of China. Some have taken such measures: the US requires domestic enterprises to move back from China by offering preferential policies; Japan suggests its firms considering moving some factories elsewhere to reduce the risk of an overly single supply chain; EU officials are talking about "strategic autonomy" and preparing to set up a fund to buy company shares. Many economists at home and abroad have commented on such moves: the US needs to pay a huge price to rebuild traditional industries requires; labor costs in the US are too high; in the age of mechanization and automation, the renewal of traditional industries will not create many jobs; moving the industrial chain out of China will increase the cost of reconstruction in other countries, with the potential risk of a poor investment environment; the most important thing is that it may lose the vast Chinese market. For these reasons, a comprehensive economic decoupling is very unlikely, but the difficulties and fluctuations in China's trade with the US and its allies are inevitable.

The Decoupling in Science and Technology is Emerging

It should be noted that this change in the US under the Trump administration is not only caused by his personal factors. Research shows that in the past decades of rapid globalization, the biggest beneficiaries are the middle and upper classes in developing countries and the high-income groups in developed countries, whereas the biggest losers are the middle and low-income groups in developed economies. Trump confronted globalization with the policy of "America First", fiercely attacking free trade and immigration. His election is a victory for the middle and lower-class whites who believe they are badly hurt by free trade. These people are also the strongest opponents of free trade and the stalwart supporters of Trump's deglobalization policy. Trump's deglobalization is not a single case. Brexit and the rise of the far right in European countries have proved that in-depth globalization will provoke populism. Due to the opposition to globalization, the areas in which the US has to work with China are narrowing.

Many international scholars have pointed out that before the COVID-19 pandemic, globalization had been strained to the limit. As a result of the pandemic, many Western countries have taken measures to curb globalization. The *Economist* even announced sadly, "Wave goodbye to the greatest era of globalization". Although deglobalization is extremely likely, it is reasonable to assume that it is only the extent of globalization that will be affected. In other words, globalization is still a general trend but may be weakened to some degree by some developed countries' deglobalization measures.

Although a complete China-US economic decoupling seems highly unlikely at present, the problem of technological decoupling has become increasingly prominent. What worries the US and other Western countries now is not only the international competitiveness of their firms and products but also their ability to ensure national security. Nowadays, the high-tech contest, which has been regarded as strategic, is still a race for world leadership in the eyes of the US. Consequently, the US has tried to take every possible measure against China's scientific and technological development, including stricter screening of foreign investment in American core technologies, a stringent examination of China's academic exchanges in the US, and the targeted increase in tariffs to reduce China's competitiveness in the key sector. It has also invested more in counter-intelligence, such as the recent ban on American exports of key products to China's artificial intelligence industry, impose a technological blockade on China. Moreover, it requires allies to collaborate. Judging from the current policy trends in the US and Europe, these measures are likely to toughen after the pandemic.

More and more people are concerned that the increasingly intense high-tech race between China and the US may lead to the division of the tech field. In the end, Europe, North America, South America, and Australia will adopt American technology and standards, while Asia, Africa, and the Middle East embrace Chinese ones. An early sign of this decoupling may be the China-US global competition for 5G standards. If the trade tension intensifies and the US tries its best to contain the Chinese market, two incompatible 5G ecosystems may take shape. The US-led system technologically supported by Silicon Valley will mainly conduct business in the highly competitive markets in developed countries. The other China-led system technologically supported by its powerful digital platform companies will focus on the markets in developing economies. Given the extent of regulation enforcement by the US, such results are not unimaginable.

Given the above situation, we must prepare well for a more difficult period of China-US relations after the coronavirus. Despite the existing social and economic problems at home, the US is unlikely to adjust its policy unless the US has a taste of its own medicine, namely, its policy proving to be counterproductive. The national security strategy of regarding China as the top competitor will persist, and a certain degree of economic decoupling and the likeliest high-tech decoupling may become reality.

特朗普与中国的贸易摩擦
——美国对"中国制造"的依赖

曹文硕（Michel Chossudovsky）[*]

近年来，美国一直通过贸易制裁威胁中国。在 2017 年 1 月特朗普政府成立之初，华盛顿不仅考虑采取对华惩罚性贸易措施，还要求"对中国的贸易行为进行调查"，重点是涉嫌侵犯美国知识产权的行为。随后，这一威胁变本加厉，"对从中国进口到美国的商品加收高额关税，取消中国公司在美国开展业务的许可证……"。接下来在 2019 年 9 月，"特朗普政府颁布对价值约 1120 亿美元的中国进口商品加征关税"。

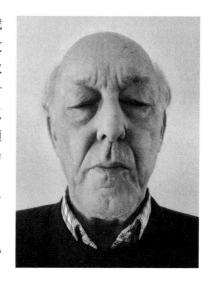

地缘政治维度

在地缘政治和战略层面上的理解至关重要，美中冲突并不仅限于双边贸易。特朗普针对中国的政治言论日益富于攻击性，其目标不言而喻是扰乱中国的"一带一路"倡议（其中包括与世界主要地区的许多伙伴国家发展贸易关系）。华盛顿认为，以欧亚经济一体化为基

础的中国"一带一路"倡议是对美国霸权利益的侵犯。托马斯·卡瓦纳在《外交官》杂志撰文称,"随着时间的流逝,'一带一路'倡议可能威胁美国第二次世界大战后的霸权根基"。美国霸权还伴随着美国对中国东海和南海战略航道的军事化,以及在中国附近地区的众多美国军事基地。

具有讽刺意味的是,特朗普的口头威胁,伴随着看似"建设性"的双边贸易谈判,最终却使美中两国在 2020 年 1 月中旬新冠肺炎疫情暴发时签署了详细而全面的第一阶段经贸协议。美国分析师认为,这份于 2020 年 1 月 15 日签署的具有历史意义的协议"有希望标志贸易摩擦开始结束"。但那并未发生。

协议签署两周后的 1 月 31 日,特朗普政府宣布对华限航、限运、限制贸易,这对中国的出口制造业产生了影响。就在世卫组织总干事 1 月 30 日宣布新冠肺炎疫情构成国际公共卫生紧急事件之后,特朗普次日立即公布了该决定。

在特朗普 1 月 31 日决定限航、限运之后,西方国家针对中国以及华裔发起了一场运动。《经济学家》报道称:"新型冠状病毒传播针对华裔的种族歧视","英国华人社区因新冠肺炎疫情暴发而遭遇种族主义"。《南华早报》报道称,"在冠状病毒暴发期间,海外华人社区正日益面临种族主义的谩骂和歧视"。而这种现象在美国随处可见。

美中贸易:美国对"中国制造"的依赖

尽管中国是关税、贸易限制以及潜在的威胁对象,但特朗普政府无法理解的是,美国严重依赖从中国进口的商品。不言而喻的是,美国是进口导向型经济,工业和制造业基础薄弱,严重依赖中国进口。尽管美国拥有金融主导地位和美元力量,但美国"实体经济"结构仍存在严重缺陷:例如标志性的工厂倒闭,以及在物质和社会基础设施上的缺陷。

这种以进口为主导的经济结构历史悠久,是美国在 20 世纪 70 年代末和 80 年代初制定的政策的结果。该政策将大部分工业基地迁至中国的"低成本"地区,包括经济特区(创建于 1979 年)、"开发区"和"特殊贸易区"(1984 年在 14 个指定的沿海城市中建立)。美国制造业的很大一部分进行了搬迁，随后又搬迁了几个高科技生产部门。

高科技

美国不再拥有高科技生产和知识产权的霸权。中国在过去的十年中巩固了自己的地位，目前在依靠自主知识产权的高科技开发和生产的几个领域处于领先地位。这不可避免地对曾经繁华的高科技产业和研究实验室摇篮——加州硅谷产生了影响。

一种相互矛盾的关系已然形成。在这种关系中，美国依赖"中国制造"的进口成品，而中国则已在包括电信和5G在内的若干高科技领域超过美国。《环球时报》2019年1月17日报道称，"所有这些案件构成了华盛顿及其盟国压制中国电信公司的大场面。华为是全球最大的电信设备制造商和全球第二大智能手机制造商，同时还生产高质量芯片。如此全面的高科技企业被指责并遭到破坏是可悲的。美国正在通过司法手段实现其政治目的"。《沃顿商学院访谈》称，"在过去二十年中，中国的技术领域发展如此迅速，以至于推翻了美国长期处于数字食物链顶端的地位。华为、微信、百度、腾讯等公司的进步正帮助中国经济以空前的速度增长并影响着全球经济。中美正在争夺5G技术的领导权，而中国科技公司似乎会赢得这场斗争的胜利"。作者丽贝卡·范宁认为，"美国需要一项能够应对中国技术进步的政策"。华盛顿所采取的"政策"似乎排除了美国"接受"中国在多个高科技领域的领先地位。

中国制造：美国零售业

想象一下，如果特朗普决定某天开始大幅减少美国的"中国制造"进口，将会发生什么。这绝对是毁灭性的，会扰乱消费经济，造成经济和金融混乱。美国大型购物中心包括大品牌在内的一大批商品都是"中国制造"。"中国制造"还主导着广泛的工业投入品、机械、建筑材料、汽车、零件和配件等的生产，更不用说美国企业集团同中国企业的广泛分包合同。

特朗普政府不理解的是美国贸易赤字最终如何使美国经济受益，

它有助于维持美国的零售经济和 GDP 增长。"中国制造"是美国零售贸易的支柱，几乎在所有主要商品类别中维持着家庭消费，包括手机、服装、鞋类、五金、医药产品、电子产品、玩具、珠宝、家用电器、食品、电视等。从中国进口是一笔数万亿美元的可观生意，它是美国巨大的利润和财富来源。从中国低成本经济体进口的消费品通常以十倍于出厂价格的零售价出售。这个过程创造了一个"附加值"，然后导致国内生产总值增加。在广泛的经济活动中，美国没有生产。生产者放弃了生产。

美国与中国的贸易逆差有助于推动以利润为导向的消费经济，而消费经济依赖中国制造的消费品。案例研究表明，中国进口产生的美国附加值 8—10 倍于进口中国商品的出厂价格。这意味着美国 GDP 增长的很大一部分归功于美国以外的生产国，即中国。没有中国的进口，美国的 GDP 增长将不可避免地受到损害。这意味着从实体经济角度看，中国是全球最大的国民经济。

中国决策者充分意识到，美国经济严重依赖"中国制造"。中国拥有超过 14 亿人口的内部市场，再加上"一带一路"倡议和蓬勃发展的全球出口市场，特朗普的威胁在某些方面就是"纸老虎"。

新型冠状病毒危机如何影响美中关系

受疫情影响，美国从中国的进口大幅下降，这对美国零售贸易的影响可能是毁灭性的。在本文中，我们应该区分以下因素：

第一，主要由具体经济因素引发的贸易中断（2020 年 1 月末至 2 月初的新冠危机造成的生产、供应链与国际运输中断）。

第二，具有政治和地缘政治性质的中断，这在很大程度上与特朗普政府声称中国应对"传播病毒"负责的指责和威胁有关。

这些指责始于 4 月。在撰写本文时，没有证据表明特朗普的指责与下面分析的 4 月商品贸易数据有关。4 月，美中贸易有恢复的趋势。

中美商贸中断

很难评估特朗普最近一波指责的影响。尽管特朗普最近威胁不断，但美国仍签署了 2020 年 1 月 15 日的美中双边经贸协议。

2018—2019 年贸易数据。美国从中国的进口额约为 4522.43 亿美元。相比之下，美国对中国的出口额约为 1066.27 亿美元，反映了美中双边贸易额相较 2018 年大幅下降。2019 年美国对中国的贸易逆差达到了惊人的 3456.17 亿美元。

2020 年 1—4 月贸易数据。2020 年的可用月度数据表明，美国从中国的每月商品进口（相对于 2019 年）大幅下降了 28.3%（2020 年的前三个月相对于 2019 年的前三个月的平均值），这主要归因于新型冠状病毒危机。

前景如何？

与 2019 年 3 月相比，2020 年 3 月美国从中国的进口下降了惊人的 36.5%。这个数字是否表明美中贸易出现了重大崩溃？在疫情之后，尽管中国的出口经济正处于正常化进程中，但包括特朗普针对中国的指责在内的政治对抗有可能导致美中双边贸易"暴跌"。

此外，根据英国《金融时报》援引的数据，新近宣布的中国对美直接投资项目价值下降了 90%，2020 年第一季度达到 2 亿美元，低于 2019 年平均每季度的 20 亿美元。"中国对美国的直接投资为 50 亿美元，较 2018 年的 54 亿美元略有下降，远低于 2016 年 450 亿美元的近期峰值，当时中国公司有更大的自由收购美国对口公司。"

然而，重要的是，根据中国海关总署 2020 年 5 月初发布的数据，中国 4 月的整体出口相对于 2019 年 4 月增长了 3.5%，全球出口额达 2003 亿美元。虽然这些数字反映了中国整体出口贸易的复苏，但中国对美国的出口在 4 月经历了 7.9% 的大幅下降，4 月对美国的出口量约为 320.604 亿美元（2019 年 4 月为 347.989 亿美元）。为弥补对美国出口的下降，中国的欧亚贸易有所增长。中国在 2020 年 4 月的进口量与 2019 年同期相比下降 14.2%，4 月份中国的贸易顺差为 453.4 亿美元。

结　语

美中关系将如何发展？美国总统新任命的国家情报总监约翰·拉

特克利夫在美国参议院听证会上明确表示：美国总统不仅没有丝毫证据就将新冠大流行归咎于中国，而且"我认为中国是目前最大的威胁行为体"，"看看新型冠状病毒和中国所起的作用，还有 5G 竞争和网络安全问题，全都指向中国"。这就是参议院委员会要求他澄清"是否会使情报程序政治化以使总统满意"时他的回答。

这一任命是否关系到美中关系的未来？5 月 21 日，约翰·拉特克利夫被提名为国家情报总监，其任务是代表特朗普白宫"反击大国的威胁"。美国国家情报总监负责监督和协调 17 个情报机构，包括中央情报局、国家安全局和联邦调查局的反情报部门。总监与白宫保持联系。其负责协调各个情报部门，但不是"情报机构"，其负责人的声明更多具有政治性质，它们将用于支持特朗普 2020 年的竞选活动。（杜鹃翻译）

原文：

Trump's Trade Friction with China
—America's Dependence on "Made in China"

Michel Chossudovsky[*]

Introduction

The US has been threatening China with trade sanctions for several years. At the outset of the Trump administration in January 2017, Washington not only envisaged punitive trade measures, it also called for "an investigation into China's trade practices" focusing on alleged violations of U. S.

---

* Michael Chossudovsky, Director, Centre for Reseach on Globalization, Montreal, Canada.

intellectual property rights. This initiative was then followed by renewed threats to "impose steep tariffs on Chinese imports into the US, rescind licenses for Chinese companies to do business in the United States..." And then in September of 2019, "The Trump administration enacted tariffs on roughly US $112 billion worth of Chinese imports".

The Geopolitical Dimension

An understanding of the geopolitical and strategic dimensions is crucial. The conflict with China is not limited to bilateral trade. President Trump's political rhetoric directed against China has become increasingly aggressive. Washington's unspoken objective is to derail China's Belt and Road Initiative (BRI) which consists in developing trade relations with a large number of partner countries in major regions of the World. China's BRI predicated on Eurasian economic integration is viewed by Washington as an encroachment on US hegemonic interests. "Over time the BRI could threaten the very foundations of Washington's post-WW Ⅱ hegemony", Thomas P. Cavanna The Diplomat. US hegemony is also coupled with US militarization of strategic waterways in the East and South China seas combined with numerous US military bases in locations within proximity of China.

In a bitter irony, the rhetorical gush of threats by president Donald Trump, was accompanied by seemingly "constructive" bilateral trade negotiations leading up to the signing of the First Phase of a detailed and comprehensive Economic and Trade Agreement between the United States and China in mid-January 2020 at the very outset of the coronavirus pandemic. According to U. S. analysts this historic Agreement signed on January 15, 2020 would "hopefully signal the beginning of the end of the trade friction". But that did not happen.

Two weeks after the signing of the Agreement, on January 31st, 2020, the Trump administration announced the curtailment of air travel with China, which was accompanied by the disruption of transportation and trade relations with China, with repercussions on China's export manufacturing sector. Trump's decision on January 31, 2020 was made public immediately following the announcement by the WHO Director General of Public Health Emergency of International Concern (PHEIC) (January 30, 2020).

And then, following Trump's January 31st decision to curtail air travel and transportation to China, a campaign was launched in Western countries against China as well ethnic Chinese. The *Economist* reported that "The coronavirus spreads racism against and among ethnic Chinese" "Britain's Chinese community faces racism over coronavirus outbreak". According to the *South China Morning Post* (Hong Kong): "Chinese communities overseas are increasingly facing racist abuse and discrimination amid the coronavirus outbreak. And this phenomenon happened all over the U. S. "

US-China Trade: America's Dependence on "Made in China"

While China is the object of tariffs, trade restrictions, not to mention veiled threats, what the Trump administration fails to comprehend is that the United States is heavily dependent on commodity imports from China. The unspoken truth is that America is an import led economy with a weak industrial and manufacturing base, heavily dependent on imports from the PRC. Despite America's financial dominance and the powers of the dollar, there are serious failures in the structure of America's "Real Economy": i. e marked by the closing down of factories as well as failures at the level of both physical and social infrastructure.

This Import-led economic structure has a long history. It was the result of US policies formulated in the late 1970s and early 1980s to delocate a large part of its industrial base to "low cost" locations in China including the Special Economic Zones (SEZ) (created in 1979) and the "development zones" or "special trading areas" (established in the 14 designated coastal cities in 1984). A large share of US manufacturing was relocated, followed by a later stage of relocation of several high technology production sectors.

High Technology

The US no longer has a hegemony in high technology production and intellectual property. In the course of the last decade, China has consolidated its position. China is now leading in several areas of high tech development and production which are dependent on Chinese owned intellectual property. This inevitably had repercussions on California's Silicone Valley, the once prosperous cradle of high tech industries and research labs.

A contradictory relationship has evolved in which the US is not only dependent on "Made in China" imported manufactured goods, China has surpassed the US in several areas of high technology including telecommunications and 5G: All the cases form a big picture in which Washington and its allies are suppressing Chinese telecom companies. Huawei is the world's largest telecom equipment maker and second largest smartphone manufacturer in the world. It also produces high-quality chips. It is pathetic that such a comprehensive high-tech enterprise Huawei is accused and undermined. The US is realizing its political purposes by judicial means. (Global Times, January 17, 2019)

According to Wharton Business School (University of Pennsylvania): "China's technology sector has grown so rapidly in the last two decades that it is pushing the United States out of its long-held position at the top of the digital food chain. Advancements by companies like Huawei, WeChat, Baidu, Tencent and others are helping the Chinese economy grow at an unprecedented rate and influencing the global economy. China and the U. S. are battling to be the leader in 5G technology, a fight it seems that Chinese tech companies are winning. " According to author Rebecca Fanning, "The U. S. needs a policy that can address China's rise in technology". It would appear that the "policy" contemplated by Washington precludes the notion of US "acceptance" of China's lead in several high technology sectors.

Made in China：Retail Trade in the US

Imagine what would happen if president Trump decided from one day to the next to significantly curtail America's "Made in China" imports. It would be absolutely devastating, disrupting the consumer economy, an economic and financial chaos. A large share of goods displayed in America's shopping malls, including major brands is "Made in China". "Made in China" also dominates the production of a wide range of industrial inputs, machinery, building materials, automotive, parts and accessories, etc. not to mention the extensive sub-contracting of Chinese companies on behalf of US conglomerates.

What the Trump Administration does not comprehend is how the US trade deficit ultimately benefits the US economy. It contributes to sustaining America's retail economy, it also sustains the growth of America's GDP. "Made in China" is the backbone of retail trade in the USA which indelibly sustains household consumption in virtually all major commodity categories from mobile phones, clothing, footwear, hardware, pharmaceutical products, electronics, toys, jewellery, household fixtures, food, TV sets, etc. Importing from China is a lucrative multi-trillion dollar operation. It is the source of tremendous profit and wealth in the US. Consumer commodities imported from China's low cost economy are often sold at the retail level ten times their factory price. This process creates a "value added" which then leads to an increase in Gross Domestic Product. In a wide range of economic activities, production does not take place in the USA. The producers have given up production.

The US trade deficit with China is instrumental in fuelling the profit driven consumer economy which relies on Made in China consumer goods. Case study suggest that China imports trigger an increase in value added in the US of 8 – 10 times the factory price of commodities imported from China. What this means is that a large share of US GDP growth is attributable to production outside the US, namely China. Without Chinese imports, the US growth of GDP would inevitably be undermined. What this signifies is that in real economy terms, China is the largest national economy Worldwide.

Chinese policy makers are fully aware that the US economy is heavily dependent on "Made in China". And with an internal market of more than 1. 4 billion people, coupled with the Belt and Road Initiative and a buoyant global export market, the veiled threats by President Trump are in some regards those of "A Paper Tiger".

How Does the Coronavirus Crisis Affect
US-China Relations

US imports from China have declined significantly as a result of the pandemic, the impacts on US retail trade are potentially devastating. In this review, we should distinguish between the following factors:

First, The disruption in trade largely triggered by concrete economic factors (production, supply lines, international transport caused by the corona crisis. This process of disruption was largely initiated in late January early February).

Second, The disruption of a political and geopolitical nature largely related to accusations and threats by the Trump administration, claiming that China is responsible for "spreading the virus".

These accusations started in April. At the time of writing, there is no evidence that president Trump's accusations have a bearing on the April commodity trade figures analyzed below. In April the tendency was towards a recovery of US-China trade.

Disruption in US-China Commodity Trade

It is difficult to assess the implications of the most recent wave of Trump accusations. Despite Trump's most recent threats, the January 15th, 2020 bilateral US-China trade agreement has been signed.

2018 – 2019 Trade Data

US imports from China were of the order of $452. 243 billion. In contrast, US exports from the US to China were of the order of $106. 627 billion reflecting a significant decline in bilateral US-China trade in relation to 2018. The US trade deficit with China in 2019 was a staggering $345. 617 billion.

January-April 2020 Trade Data

The available monthly figures for 2020 suggest a substantial decline in (monthly) US commodity imports from China (in relation to 2019): A 28. 3% decline (average over first three months of 2020 in relation to first 3 months of 2019), largely attributable to the coronavirus crisis.

What are the Prospects?

The decline of US imports from China in the month of March was of a staggering 36. 5% in relation to March 2019. Does this figure indicate a significant collapse in US-China trade? While China's export economy is in the process of normalization in the wake of the China pandemic, the political confrontations including the accusations directed against China by president Trump could potentially lead to a "slump" in US-China bilateral trade.

Moreover, according to figures quoted by the the Financial Times, the value of newly announced Chinese direct investment projects into the US has fallen by about 90% : US $200 million in the first quarter of 2020, down from an average of US $2 billion per quarter in 2019. "Chinese direct investment into the US stood at US $5 billion, a slight drop from US $5. 4

billion in 2018 and well off a recent peak of US $45 billion in 2016, when Chinese companies were much more free to acquire US counterparts."

What is significant, however, is that China's overall exports (dollars) in April rose by 3.5% (in relation to April 2019), according to data from China's General Administration of Customs released in early May. In April 2020, in dollar terms China's exports (Worldwide) amounted to US $200.3 billion. While these figures reflect a recovery of China's overall export trade, China's exports to the US in April experienced a significant decline, namely 7.9%. Exports to the US in April were of the order of the order of 32,060.4 million (compared to 34,798.9 million in April 2019). In contrast, compensating for the decline in exports to the US, China's Eurasian trade has picked up. China's imports in April 2020 fell 14.2% in relation to the same period in 2019. China's trade surplus for the month of April was US $45.34 billion.

Concluding Remarks

How will US-China relations evolve? The US president is not only blaming China for the corona pandemic without a shred of evidence, his newly appointed Director of National Intelligence (DNI) Rep. John Ratcliffe stated unequivocally at the US Senate confirmation hearing: "I view China as the greatest threat actor right now" "Look with respect to COVID-19 and the role China plays; the race to 5G; cybersecurity issues: all roads lead to China," he told the panel. To which the Senate Committee asked him to clarify: "whether he would politicize the intelligence process to keep the president happy."

Does this appointment have a bearing on the future of US-China relations? On May 21, Rep Ratcliffe was nominated as DNI with a mandate to "counter threats from great powers" on behalf of the Trump Whitehouse. The Director of the DNI oversees and coordinates 16 intelligence bodies, including the CIA, the National Security Agency (NSA), and the

FBI's counterintelligence division. The head of the DNI has links to the White House. While it coordinates the various Intel entities, it is not an "intelligence agency". Declarations from the head of DNI are more of political nature. They will be used in support of Trump's 2020 election campaign.

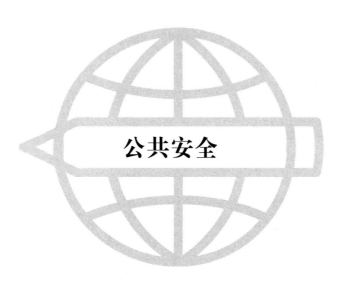

公共安全

从新型冠状病毒说开去

维克多·拉林 （Viktor Larin）*

如今，许多媒体都在写文章，许多人都在公开评论，说这次新型冠状病毒正在改变世界。对此我不认同。事实上，早在这次疫情之前世界便已开始发生剧变。这次变化最大的特点是西方国家保守数百年的政治、经济，以及意识形态层面的统治地位正逐渐让步给东方世界。中国在全球范围的部署迫使许多西方政客从苏联解体后的美梦中猛然惊醒，环顾四周，突然发现自己的王朝即将走向末路。而且，这个雄心勃勃、不屈不挠，发

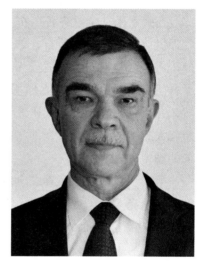

展速度在西方世界看来无法想象的中国甚至与突然振作的俄罗斯结伴，两国意在共同打破西方统治，重塑世界秩序，这些是西方政客随手摆弄的工具，同时也无比珍贵。

这场与新冠肺炎疫情的较量将东西方权力交叠的进程暴露给了全球民众。西方世界在经历这些变化时显得痛苦不堪，一些西方国家秉持的所谓普世价值观也好像走到了尽头。当生命危在旦夕时，这些价值观将很快被抛在脑后。当关乎人类命运时，很少有人会想起自由、民主等价值观。但总的来说，不论是从组织层面还是从道德层面，西

* 维克多·拉林，俄罗斯科学院通讯院士，俄罗斯科学院远东分院副院长。

方国家对这次不是特别致命的疫情的反应显然是不够的。

与此相比，亚洲国家为应对包括这次疫情在内的突发事件做了更充分的准备。在这些地方，"民主"概念的地位要次于传统的社会组织架构。西方世界担心，国际社会会将中国的政治模式视为西方选举民主的替代方案，并为前者投"信任票"，其他国家完全可以循着这条新路寻求和平、繁荣和现代化。在与新型冠状病毒的斗争中，中国向全世界展示了一种管理社会、解决极端问题的有效体系，必将吸引大量支持者和跟随者。如今，中国已逐步摆脱因疫情导致的经济停滞，这将是另一大有力佐证。

在我看来，全世界各国都应该从这次疫情中吸取一些宝贵的经验教训。第一，据专家所言，这次新型冠状病毒是从自然界中变异而来的。正是因为人们无法适应亲手造成的环境变化才产生了这次疫情。大自然再次展示了它不愿屈服于人类的一面。为此，人类应保护自然，并持续对大自然开展研究。若非这次新冠肺炎疫情，人们也不会想起大自然的真正价值，即晴空、蓝天、绿植、碧水和自由沟通所带来的愉悦。

第二，新型冠状病毒在全球传播也揭示了全球化的利弊。所有国家都在一条船上。但事实是，有人等着救生员来施救，有人有救生圈，有人被直升机救出，剩下的人只能靠自己。酒神节过后，有人变得更加富有，而有人注定要饿死。这是又一次大考，考验政府和政治家的能力，考验国家和人民的团结，考验友谊也考验敌对。不是所有人都能挺过这一关。像历史上任何一次危机一样，总有一些普通人展现了人类最宝贵的品质，如善良、勇气、毅力和人道主义。还有一些人仗着一点权势行小人之事。

第三，为了赢得这场在全球范围内全面展开的混合战争，我们首先应该投资的不是武器，而是研究人类及其不断变化的环境。不幸的是，医学界当时未就这次由自然界主导的冲击做好准备。科学家预料到可能会出现与这次新型冠状病毒相似的病毒，但无法为此做好准备。在此次新型冠状病毒暴发6个月以后，目前最好的"解药"仍是"待在家中别乱跑"。世界各国都遇到了相同的麻烦，只有高效协作才能应对这一问题。不光在医疗领域，我们必须在各领域开展国际合作。

疫情在俄罗斯流行以后，一个显著的结果是，政府官员突然意识到了医疗专业和医药产业的重要性。他们随即开始将更多的资金投向医学，并公开谈论医学的重要性。医生和科学家开始被请上了电视。所以，这次疫情至少带来了一点好处，即医务工作者的声誉和地位得到了提高。

新型冠状病毒从何而来并不重要。重要的是，西方国家秉持着"在爱与战争中一切都是公平的"原则，正尝试利用这次疫情作为又一手段，维系其世界影响力和统治地位。西方国家起诉中国政府"故意隐瞒信息，掩盖新型冠状病毒的威胁"。这一行为尽冷嘲热讽之能事，看起来很愚蠢，同时也展示了特朗普的无能。我觉得是时候控诉美国了，控诉他们金融监管不力、公司管理违规、建立"影子"银行、金融体系崩溃导致 2008 年国际金融危机。但是特朗普死皮赖脸，无所作为。一方面，他要应对国内的政治问题；另一方面，他在制造舆论宣传，企图为一系列措施加码，阻止中国扩大其全球影响力。美国认为，人类命运共同体理念无法维系其统治地位，将不惜一切手段与之斗争。

此次新冠肺炎疫情也是对中俄两国间的友谊和信任的一次考验。当疫情在中国暴发，中俄两国的边境被关闭，中国的感染者入境俄罗斯时，有人尝试发起新一轮的中国威胁论。但是这些尝试很快就销声匿迹了，因为俄罗斯国内的新型冠状病毒并不是中国人带来的，而是来自欧洲。我不清楚俄罗斯采取了何种机制，但在这特殊时期，为了防止病毒传入俄罗斯境内，即使是再小的漏洞也会被俄方熟练且迅速地关闭。疫情刚暴发时，俄罗斯曾对中国施以援助。现在，中国从疫情中慢慢恢复过来了，转而帮助了俄罗斯。我想，这大概就是"战略伙伴关系"、两国相互信任和两国民众间无私友谊的真正含义。

这场疫情很快就会结束。那些准备更加充分、应对更加得当的国家是这场全球危机的最终赢家。

但是，我坚信，美国还会从其武器库中搬出更多的花样用以阻止中国提升其在世界上的影响力。（董方源翻译）

原文：

Coronavirus and around

Viktor Larin*

Today, many speak and write that coronavirus is changing the world. I do not agree. The world began to change dramatically long before the epidemic. The quintessence of this change is the loss by the West of centuries of political, economic and—most importantly—ideological dominance over the East. The global march of China has forced many politicians in the West, who have greatly relaxed after the collapse of the USSR, to shake themselves, look around and suddenly see that their resting on their laurels is coming to an end. Moreover, this incomprehensible, ambitious and unyielding China even more made friends with unexpectedly perked up Russia, and together they intend to remake the world of Western domination which is so dear and convenient for these politicians.

The fight against the epidemic of coronavirus only bare, exposed ongoing processes to the public. She showed how painfully the Western world is experiencing these changes, which demonstrate the ephemeral nature of some of its supposedly universal values, which are instantly forgotten when your own life is at stake. Few people recall such values as freedom or democracy when it comes to human beings. But in general, the reaction of the West to a not so deadly epidemic is clearly inadequate from the point of view of or-

* Viktor Larin, Corresponding Academician, Russian Academy of Sciences; Vice President, Russian Academy of Sciences Far Eastern Branch.

ganizing the fight against it, and from a moral point of view.

But she also demonstrated that Asian civilizations, where the concept of "democracy" is secondary to a traditional social organization, are better prepared to deal with such misfortunes as the epidemic. The West's fears that the international community will see in the CCP's model an alternative to Western electoral democracy and give it a "credit of confidence" to develop a new path to peace, prosperity and modernity that other countries can follow have every reason. In its fight against the coronavirus, China introduced the world to an effective system of managing society and solving extreme problems, which will have adherents and followers. His exit from the strip of economic stagnation will be another proof of the effectiveness of this system.

It seems to me that the world should learn some important lessons from current events. The first, according to experts, the current epidemic is an environmentally determined problem. It arose because people could not adapt to environmental changes that they themselves created. The nature once again demonstrated its unwillingness to obey, recalled the importance of caring for it and its continuous study. If there were no epidemic of coronavirus, it should have been invented to remind humanity of the real values it possesses: clear air, blue skies, green forests, clearwater and the happiness of open communication.

Second lesson. The spread of coronavirus across the planet has clearly demonstrated the pros and cons of globalization. We are really all in the same boat. But the only truth is that someone will be followed by rescuers, someone has a lifebuoy, someone is evacuated by helicopter, and the rest have to rely only on themselves. After all this bacchanalia, someone will become much richer, and someone is destined to die of hunger. This is another test of the quality of governments and politicians, states and peoples, friends and enemies. Not everyone can stand it. As in any crisis situation, there are ordinary people who show the best human qualities: humanism, kindness, courage, stamina, and there are figures from false pedestals that behave like small people.

Lesson Three. To win the hybrid war, which is already in full swing on the planet, one must invest first, not in armaments, but in the study of man and his changing environment. Unfortunately, medical science was not ready for such a blow from nature. Scientists assumed the appearance of something similar to the current COVID-19, but could not prepare for it. Almost six months after the outbreak of coronavirus, the main cure for it remains "staying home." The trouble is common, and it is only possible to deal with it effectively together. International cooperation in this is imperative. And not only in the field of medical research.

One noticeable consequence of the epidemic in Russia is that officials suddenly realized the importance of medicine and the importance of the medical profession. They began to invest much more money than before into medicine, talk about medical science. Scientists and doctors began to be invited to television. Maybe in increasing the prestige and status of a medical worker there will be at least one positive result of the epidemic.

It doesn't matter where the coronavirus came from. It is important that the Western world is trying to use the epidemic as another tool to maintain its dominant position, its influence in the world. It doesn't matter where the coronavirus came from. It is important that the Western world is trying to use the epidemic as another tool to maintain its dominant position, its influence in the world, following the principle "all is fair in love and war." Filing a lawsuit against the Chinese government for "sheltering information about the dangers of coronavirus", of course, looks silly, seems to be the height of cynicism and recognition President Trump own incompetence. Then it's time to sue the United States for failures in financial regulation, violations in the field of corporate governance, the creation of a "shadow" banking system, the collapse of which gave rise to the global financial and economic crisis of 2008. But Trump does nothing for nothing. On the one hand, he is solving his domestic political problems, on the other, he is making another propaganda move, adding a link to the chain of Washington actions aimed at preventing the further growth of China's authority and popularity in the world. America does not see its future in the community with a shared future for mankind, and will fight against it by any means.

For Russian-Chinese relations, the coronavirus epidemic has also become a test of friendship and trust. When an epidemic erupted in China, borders were closed, there were attempts to initiate a new wave of China-phobia. But they quickly faded away. The virus was brought to Russia not from China, but from Europe. I don't know what mechanisms were used, but even a narrow loophole for the virus to penetrate from China to Russia was very quickly and skillfully closed. Russia helped China, China, recovering from the virus, helped Russia. This, probably, is one of the meanings of "strategic partnership", mutual trust between our countries and disinterested friendship between people.

The epidemic will end soon. The winner is the one who is better prepared, who is better than others to cope with the consequences of this global insanity.

I am sure that there is more than one piece in Washington's arsenal that will be used to stop China's triumphant progress to improve international influence.

拥有人类共同未来的共同体

——流行病对世界的影响与合作

斯捷潘·梅西奇（Stjepan Mesic）[*]

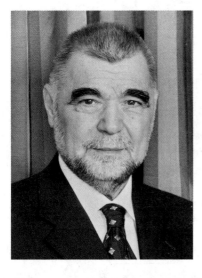

目前的新型冠状病毒危机席卷了整个世界，造成了人类巨大的伤痛，也使全球经济前景暗淡。没有哪个国家能够独善其身，除非所有的国家都平安度过危机，而如果没有全球的、地区的和全国的合作，这几乎不可能实现。如果有什么我们能从这场卫生的危机中学到的教训，那就是这个世界应该团结在一起，对于新冠病毒肺炎只做出一国自己的应对既不能解决危机，也不能让世界为下一次到来的流行病做好适当的准备。全球对此做出回应，则会对应对流行病提供符合逻辑的出路，但是在这个全世界人民的艰难时刻，这看上去还未确定，甚至是不确定的。

美国是世界领先的经济体，也是军事上的超级大国，但却暂停了对世界卫生组织的资助，在很多国家看来，这是对于这一组织在全球所发挥的作用的不恰当的打击，并且削弱了全球协作对这一史无前例的健康危机做出回应的机会。美国的软实力在于其塑造其他国家偏好的能力，而由于美国政府的这一行动，美国的软实力遭到了严重的打

＊ 斯捷潘·梅西奇，克罗地亚前总统。

击。在这次流行病危机期间，美国的道德权威及其全球作用因其自己的政府而受到了强烈的震动。

世界卫生组织天然的职责就是领导协调各国（对健康危机）的应对，应该得到联合国和世界各国的支持。全球性的流行病可能威胁到国际和平与稳定，联合国安理会的成员国应该迅速做出反应，采取措施，联合国应该致力于对此做出全球层面上的应对。

与其他国家和国际机构合作来制订一个全球计划，应自己的公民的需要承担责任来抗击病毒，美国政府并不认为这是自己应发挥的作用。在这种情况下，其他全球大国——欧盟、中国和俄罗斯应该领导全球更为公开地支持世界卫生组织，并给予其更多的财政资源。

欧盟明白世界卫生组织作为重要的全球组织在艰难应对新型冠状病毒危机的过程中享有强大的公信力。欧盟对于正在发生中的新型冠状病毒危机所做出的反应并不快，而是更为缓慢，更为渐进，因为在其历史上，欧盟从未遭遇这样的流行病，这将使其经济停滞。在危机的最初几周中，欧盟一直遭到批评，因为其成员国之间不够团结，在延缓病毒传播的健康合作方面很脆弱，但是现在欧盟显示出了应对这样一场危机的经济实力。新冠病毒肺炎以及对希腊的救助显示出欧洲北部和南部的分歧仍然存在，但是这一次欧元区的决策者们决定为 19 个使用单一货币的国家建立 5000 亿欧元的基金，以解决危机。

这对欧盟来说是和平时期最大的挑战，欧盟深知应对这场流行病需要全球对此做出回应，采取全球的行动，进行全球的协调，这对挽救人们的生命、对经济增长和世界稳定至关重要。

中国是最早遭到新冠病毒肺炎打击的国家之一，中国强烈支持世界卫生组织和联合国作为全球应对这场流行病的核心机构，强调全球合作的必要性。中国已经帮助了世界上许多的国家，向其提供医疗捐助，组织重要医疗设备的生产和出口，尽管中国的武汉曾经封城近三个月。

如果在未来的岁月中，这个世界的秩序仍建立在权力政治、单边主义和国际机构的弱化的基础上，那么全球合作几乎不可能实施。此时此刻，中国是唯一有人类共同命运这一观念的国家，这样的观念将有助于在全球性流行病挑战世界稳定这样的挑战发生之际提供长远的解决之道。

最近习近平主席与联合国秘书长安东尼奥·古特雷斯交谈时又提到了这一概念，将在新的历史时期在全世界树立人类共同体的理念，支持人类共同理想和美好追求。

习近平主席于 2013 年提出了构建人类命运共同体的倡议。2017年，在第 71 届联合国大会上通过一项关于"联合国与全球经济治理"的决议，将中国"共商、共建、共享"理念融入其中，这将有助于世界在结构上做好准备从国家层面、地区层面和全球层面应对未来任何的健康危机。

思考人类的利益，而不仅仅是利润目标，希望国际关系能够通过这样的方式得到提升。（毛悦翻译）

原文：

The Community with a Shared Future for Mankind

—Impact of the Pandemic on the World and Cooperation

Stjepan Mesic[*]

The current coronavirus crisis hit the whole world, causing immense human suffering and grave prospects for the global economy. And no country could be safe unless all countries are safe whtoh is hardly possible without global, regional and national cooperation. If there is any lesson to be learned already now from the sanitary crisis, it should be that the world is globally

---

[*] Stjepan Mesic, Former President, Croatia.

connected and only national answer on the COVID-19 will not solve the crisis nor prepare the world for next pandemic properly.

The global response provides a logical way for respond to epidemics but in this hard time for people of the whole world it appears pretty undetermined and even uncertain.

The USA, leading economy and military superpower, frozen its funds for the WHO that has been seen in many countries as an unappropriated attack on the global role of this organisation and weakening chances for global response on this unprecedented health crisis. America's soft power that rests on the ability to shape the preferences of others, has been hardly hit with that move. In this pandemic America's moral authority and its global role has been strongly shaken by its own government.

The WHO natural role is to take the lead in coordinating a national response and should be supported by all countries and by the United Nations. The Security Council members should act quickly and adopt approach that global pandemic may threaten international peace and stability how could the UN work on global response.

In the situation when the United States administration does not see its role as a work with other states and global institutions to develop a global plan and take responsibility for fighting the virus with the needs of its citizens. Globally, other global powers European Union, China and Russia should take global leadership supporting more openly the WHO and give it more financial resources.

The European Union understand the WHO as an important global organisation in managing the corona crisis with strong credibility. Brussels reaction on the on-going coronavirus crisis has not been quick but slower and more gradual because never in its history the Union was faced with such kind of pandemic that should halting of its economy.

In the first weeks of crisis Brussels has been criticised for lacking solidarity among member states and fragile health cooperation in slowing the spread of the virus but now the EU shows it has economic of financial capacity to respond to a crisis of such proportion. The COVID-19, as well as bailout of Greece, has shown that division among north and south in Europe is present but this time eurozone policymakers decided to solve the crisis establishing the fund of 500 billion euros for 19 countries that use single currency.

This is the greatest peacetime challenge to the EU that is deeply aware the pandemic needs a global response, global action and coordination that is vital for lives of people, for economy growth and for the world stability.

China, that was one of the first countries hit by COVID-19 strongly supports the WHO and the UN as a central organisation in defining global approach to the pandemic stressing that global cooperation is needed. China has helped many countries in the world with medical donation as well with its ability to organise production of vital medical equipment and export, though it had lockdown for three months in Wuhan.

The global cooperation hardly could be implemented if order in the world in next decades will continue to be based on old pattern of power politics, unilateralism and weakening of global institutions. At the moment China is only country that have a concept of a shared destiny for humanity that could be useful in providing long term answer on challenge of the global pandemic to the world stability.

Recently President Xi Jinping talked again about the concept with Secretary General of UN António Guterres who supported the common ideal and good pursuit of mankind, elevating the ideas of the common people in the world in a new historical period.

China launched the concept of building community with a shared future for mankind in 2013 and the 71st session of the UN General Assembly passed a resolution on "United Nations and global economic governance", incorporating China's concept of "Consultation, contribution and shared benefits".

Implementation of this concept could help the world to be structurally prepared to manage any future health crisis nationally, regionally and globally.

Hope the international relations will be upgraded in that way that thinks about the interests of humanity not only about profit goals.

新冠肺炎疫情期间的公共安全

杨　博（Yang Peou）*

新冠肺炎疫情造成的国际公共安全挑战

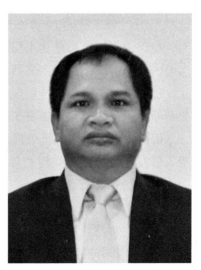

关于此次疫情暴发，我个人认为国际公共安全面临五大挑战。第一，此次疫情对世界秩序造成了冲击。毫无疑问，新冠病毒肺炎促使我们重新思考对安全构成威胁的因素。同其他类似疾病相比，新冠病毒肺炎传播速度更快、范围更广。尽管有世界卫生组织的指导方针，各国仍然各自采取了独立举措，包括实施隔离、关闭边境、停止国际运输，推迟或取消文化体育活动等。即便如此，这些政策似乎也没能阻止感染与死亡人数的上升。根据世界实时统计数据显示，截止到 2020 年 6 月 12 日，全世界共有 7597347 例感染病例，死亡人数达 423846 人。在新冠病毒肺炎感染病例最多的五个国家当中，美国位居首位，其次是巴西、俄罗斯、印度与英国。

第二，肇始于美国总统唐纳德·特朗普，各国相互指责对方制造了病毒的行为，加剧了国际对抗，并有可能导致超级大国之间的又一次冷战。事实真相遭到压制，透明度缺失，荒诞的主张与彻头彻尾虚

* 杨博，柬埔寨皇家科学院秘书长。

假、充满误导性的新闻在一些国家蔓延开来，引发了恐慌，并使得预防举措失效。2020年面临连任竞选的美国总统特朗普因其应对疫情的方式失当而备受诟病，他怪罪中国试图掩盖疫情的暴发，并指责世卫组织未能追究北京方面的责任，称世卫组织"唯中国马首是瞻""是中国的傀儡"。对此，中国外交部部长王毅指责美国在新型冠状病毒问题上散播"阴谋与谎言"，加剧了两国之间的紧张局势。他表示，美国已经感染上了某种"政治病毒"，这种病毒迫使一些政客一再攻击中国。

第三，反恐合作的机会将会丧失。新冠肺炎疫情越过诸如"基地"组织与ISIS这样的恐怖组织，攫取了各国政府与民众的关注，而这类恐怖组织恰恰是从不稳定与混乱中吸取养分从而壮大，并将在当前的形势下继续恐怖主义活动。此外，世界各地的紧张局势都在激化，已不仅仅局限于战争地区。在巴西、印度、科索沃、马拉维、南非与菲律宾群岛等地都爆发了抗议活动。

第四，种族主义与排外情绪正在抬头。随着病毒的传播，针对亚裔人群及亚裔长相的种族主义与排外态度在其他国家普遍存在，因被指责为疫情的始作俑者，很多人遭到排斥。与此同时，一名叫作乔治·弗洛伊德的黑人被杀，又引发了美国近期的一次大骚乱，这又使得特朗普政府投入了大量金钱与精力来反对这一种族主义。

第五，随着经济不确定性的增加，世界经济正遭遇快速衰退。全球各大银行与投资公司正为此做好准备。实体经济也面临前所未有的压力，大量中小企业倒闭。最先因疫情受损的是航空部门，接下来是旅游业、体育与文化活动。边境关闭阻碍了贸易。一场连锁反应导致几乎所有的经济类别都遭受了螺旋式下跌。各地失业率上升。经济复苏需要政府发挥更大的作用。在为各国政府的努力提供资金支持上，国际金融机构至关重要。

公共安全确保了世界的共同发展

在特朗普政府的推动下，美国更加无视联合国宪章原则所倡导的积极共存。与此同时，美国国内的共和党与民主党之争持续升温；最终，在疫情肆虐下，这不仅造成了美国国内的不良后果，也加深了国际社会的忧虑。

新型冠状病毒尚无药可解，它夺去了成千上万美国人的性命，也摧毁了美国的经济。一些专家认为，疫情大大降低了特朗普对抗乔·拜登的可能性，因此他需要尽一切可能攻击他的政治对手，比如嘲笑拜登是"昏昏欲睡的乔"。

对于上述问题，我认为，世界应做好防范疫情的准备，这包括重塑医疗卫生部门。进一步讲，我们应建立信任以达成全球和谐。在安全与和平社会的共同愿景下建立关系网络并开展合作，已迫在眉睫。考虑到当前环境下全球援助至关重要，所有国家，特别是最不发达的国家应该获得外国援助，通常是粮食安全与公共卫生方面的援助。

为今天的公共安全负责，加大公共安全领域的公共产品投入

我们应着眼于四个因素来考虑对当今公共安全负有责任的参与者。第一，我们需要反思历史上曾经暴发过的流行病。世界范围内暴发过数次疫情，那么谁应当对这些事件负责值得思考。比如黑死病，于 1347 年被黑海上的船只带到了欧洲，袭击了亚洲与欧洲。在随后的五年间，这场疾病造成了两千万人死亡。在当时，似乎并没有对这一事件的合理解释。可以说，没有有效的工具来确定造成此次事件的真正原因，直到 19 世纪末法国生物学家发现细菌。不过，上述疾病的暴发并不是欧洲唯一的一场疫情。

现在，让我们回顾一下百年之前暴发的疫情，比如 1918 年的西班牙流感。后来暴发的这场疾病成为 20 世纪最致命的疫情，全世界有五千万人死亡、超过 5 亿人感染。流感最早是在美军中发现的。成千上万的美国士兵参加了第一次世界大战并被部署到世界各地参战，导致了流感在全球尤其是欧洲的传播。没有人声称对此负责，也没有人因造成了这场毁灭性的流行病而受到指责。

第二，现代技术为疾病传播提供了可能的路径。疾病识别可能需要时间来找出致病原因，发现其造成的后果。比如，在所谓的疾病暴

发初期，如果没有准确的信息与实验室的检测结果，主管部门很难立即向公众发出警告。在此情况下，受感染人群会扩散开来，被各种交通工具带至不同的地点。交通工具现代化程度越高，疾病传播的速度就越快。

第三，疾病预防及知识的局限性。在没有疾病发生的严重警告下，人们和有关当局或许不会认真采取预防措施，甚至不会相信有重大疾病暴发，这种情况一般都会发生。人们继续不当一回事，还有不符合政府规定措施的公共行为也会导致感染的进一步增加。大家认为这种情况最有可能发生在世界上的发展中国家，但即便是像意大利这样的欧洲富国，也难以在新型冠状病毒暴发之初说服其民众认识到疾病的严重性。

第四，也是非常重要的一点，是有限的医疗响应以及防范计划的局限性也可能造成疾病在全球的迅速传播。

因此，为了响应并推动该领域内公共产品的投入，我们应考虑以下三大举措。首先，最重要的是提高全球每个公民的卫生意识与知识。这有助于预防感染的发生，也能在时间上减缓疾病的传播与感染。其次，为那些最需要的国家就卫生相关问题提供医疗支持，也将有助于控制不安全事件的发生。最后，针对每一次暴发的高效防范计划也应纳入考量，并在急需时采取有效行动。这些措施将大大有助于在疾病及其他任何事件的暴发前、暴发时及暴发后作出及时而迅速的反应，从而有助于重塑并稳定公共安全。

推动公共新安全

唐纳德·特朗普总统已经在声明中表示"美国优先的外交政策正在运行"。从战略上讲，"美国优先"是种自私自利的做法，人们不认为这是一种能有效控制美国国内的新型冠状病毒的举措。在其总统任期的领导下，某种意义上的非政治现实主义无助于特朗普政府重筑信心。特朗普正在拿新型冠状病毒的诞生地大做文章，推卸责任，这就是最好的例证。尽管如此，他并没有大力加强任何国际合作以应对疫情。相反，他过于关注中国在世界秩序中的突出作用。另外，自从他对即将到来的 2020 年 11 月举行的总统选举表示担忧后，他就表现出了强硬的反应。显而易见的是，皮尤研究中心的一项调查结果显示，美国的几大盟友，即澳大利亚、加拿大和韩国，对特朗普干预世界事务缺乏公众信心。这对美国外交政策的成果而言可能是个关键的暗示。因此，疫情期间发生的这些事不过是中国不可避免且相应地达到了在现实中担起领导责任的历史转折点。（杨莉翻译）

原文：

Public Security During the COVID-19 Pandemic

Yang Peou[*]

Challenges of International Public Security by the Pandemic

Related to the outbreak of this pandemic, I personally see five main challenges of the international public security. First, it causes impacts on the world order. Certainly, COVID-19 causes us to reconsider what composes security threats. COVID-19 spreads more quickly and expansively than other similar diseases, and despite World Health Organization (WHO) guidelines, each country has taken its own independent measures, including implementing quarantines, closing borders, preventing international transportation, and delaying or canceling sport and cultural events, among others;

---
* YANG Peou, Secretary-General, Royal Academy of Cambodia.

nevertheless, these policies seem not to prevent the number of cases and deaths from increasing. According to Worldometer, there are 7597347 coronavirus cases in the world, with the total death of 423846 as if June 12, 2020. USA ranks first, followed by Brazil, Russia, India, and UK, in the top five countries of COVID-19 cases.

Second, it increases the international confrontation by accusing one another of creating the virus, especially the ignition by US President Donald Trump, which can lead to another cold war between the superpowers. Transparency has been absent because facts are being suppressed, wild assertions and outright false and misleading news are spreading in some countries, causing panic and making preventive measures ineffective. US President Donald Trump, who faces re-election this year and has been criticized for his handling of the pandemic, has blamed China for trying to cover up the outbreak and has accused the WHO of failing to hold Beijing to account, calling WHO as "China-centric" and "a puppet of China". In response to this, China's Foreign Minister Wang Yi has accused the US of spreading "conspiracies and lies" about the coronavirus, ratcheting up tensions between the two nations. He said the US has been infected by a "political virus" that compels some politicians to repeatedly attack China.

Third, the opportunity of anti-terrorism cooperation will be lost. This new pandemic has captured the attention of governments and citizens more than terrorist groups as al-Qaeda and ISIS who thrive off of instability and chaos but will continue their terrorism in the current climate. Also, tensions are already flaring around the world, and not just in war zones. Protests have broken out from Brazil, India, Kosovo, Malawi, South Africa, and the Philippines.

Fourth, racism and xenophobia are on the rise. As the virus spread, racist and xenophobic attitudes toward people of Asian descent and appearance have been prevalent in other countries. Many have been ostracized after being accused as the originators of the pandemic. Meanwhile, a recent riot occurring in the US due to the killing of one black man George Floyd has cost Donald Trump's administration a lot of money and effort to fight against this racism.

Fifth, world economy is plummeting as economic uncertainty is growing. Global banks and investment firms are bracing themselves. The real economy is also under unprecedented strain with massive numbers of SME businesses closing down. The aviation sector was the first to be damaged by the pandemic, and after it, tourism, sports, and cultural events. Closed borders hindered commerce. A chain reaction resulted in a downward spiral in almost all economic categories. Unemployment rose everywhere. Economic recovery will require an increased state role to redress suffering. International financial institutions will be essential to funding these efforts.

Public Security Protect and Secure the Common Development of the World

The administration of Trump is pushing the US to deeply involve in disregarding positive co-existence of the United Nations based on the principle of charters of the UN. Meanwhile, the stark challenge between the Republican and Democratic parties keeps rising in the US; therefore, it is not only constituted American adverse results but also the international concerns amid unrestrained pandemic.

The Coronavirus which is remained unresolved has claimed thousands of American lives and devastated the US economy. Some experts believe that the pandemic provides fewer possible choices for Trump to battle with Joe Biden so that he needs to attack his political opponent in any way possible, such as mocking Biden as "Sleepy Joe".

Regarding the aforementioned, I think that the world should be in a state of preparedness against the pandemic, including reshaping the medical health sectors. Furthermore, we should build up trust for the global harmonization. Networking and cooperation with a common vision of a safe and peaceful community, are compelling. Given that global assistance is vital in the current context, all of the countries, particularly the least developed ones should be supported by foreign aid, usually in the form of food security and public health.

Responsibility for Today's Public Security and Improve the Input of Public Goods in the Field of Public Security

To consider the actors responsible for today's public security, we shall look at four factors. First, we need to consider historical pandemics. There have been many disease outbreaks worldwide and who would consider being responsible for these incidents. The Black Death, for instance, brought to Europe in 1347 by ships from the Black Sea, striking Europe and Asia. It caused more than 20 million death over the following five years. During that time there seemed to be no rational explanation for this incident. It can be said that there were no efficient tools to figure out what really the causes of incidents; until the end of the 19th century, the French biologist discovered the germ. Though, the above-mentioned outbreak is not the only disease pandemic in Europe.

Now, take the look at the last 100-year outbreak, such as the 1918 Spanish flu. The latter disease caused the deadliest pandemic of the 20th century with more than 50 million death worldwide and more than 500 million people infected. It was identified firstly in the US military personnel 1918. Hundreds and thousands of US soldiers engaged the WWI and traveled to deploy for war and contributed to the global spread of flu, especially in Europe. Nobody claimed to be responsible, nor to be accused of this devastating pandemics.

Secondly, modern technology enables the means of disease transmission. Disease identification may need time to figure out the cause and the consequences. At the primary occurrence of the so-called disease outbreak, it would be hard for the competent sector to issue such an immediate warning to the civilians without any accurate information or test result from the laboratory, for example. In this case, the spreading of infected humans would happen and be brought to different locations through various transport means. The more modern transport means are, the fastest spreading of disease infection is.

The third factor should be considered the limitation of disease prevention and knowledge. This may happen generally, while there is no critical warning of the disease occurrence, people and certain relevant authorities may not seriously conduct preventive measures or even believe such a serious disease outbreak. People's continuous response and public behavior that do not conform to measures stipulated by governments, also lead to an increase in incidents of infection. This could be considered to be most likely happened in the developing countries worldwide, but several rich countries in Europe like Italy are also hard to convince its people at the beginning of the COVID-19 outbreak.

Last but not least, limited medical response and its efficiency preparedness plans could contribute to the fast disease spreading globally.

Therefore, in order to respond to and promote the input of public goods in such a field, we shall take into consideration three main measures. First and foremost, increase health awareness and knowledge to every citizen globally. This will help to avoid the infection incident and also to slow down in the time of the disease spreading and infection. In addition, medical supports to health issues especially in those countries who need the most, contribute to controlling unsecured incidents. Finally, effective preparedness plans for every outbreak need to considerably take into account and take action efficiently in a time of need. These could considerably contribute to a fast and immediate response on time prior, during, and after the disease outbreak or any other incident and consequently, help to reshape and stabilize the public security.

Promote the New Public Security

President Donald Trump has expressed his national security strategy statement, "America First foreign policy in action". Strategically, American First is related to a self-interested approach which is believed not to be an effective implication to control the Coronavirus outbreak in the USA sense of non-political realism has not helped the administration of Trump restore confidence under his presidential leadership. As an illustration, Trump is playing his blame game over the birth of the Coronavirus pandemic; however, he has not greatly strengthened any cooperative international response. Rather, Trump has got over concerned with the prominent roles of China in the world order. Also, Trump has expressed his hard-line reaction since he has shown concern about the possibility of the short-coming presidential election damage to be held in November 2020. Evidently, the result from a survey undertaken by Pew Research Center has revealed that there has been a lack of global public confidence in his world-affair intervention among democratic US allies, namely Australia, Canada, and South Korea. It can be a pivotal implication for ensuring American diplomatic policy achievement. As a result, what happens, amid the pandemic, is that China unavoidably and accordingly reaches her historical turning point of the leading role of reality.

后疫情时代，疫情和气候变化合作模式应如何深刻调整？

史蒂夫·霍华德（Steve Howard）*

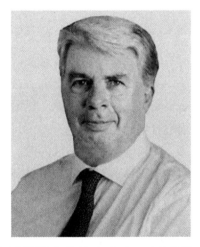

这一切的结局如何？就目前来看，不太乐观。

毫无疑问，世界终将驯服并战胜新型冠状病毒，全球经济也将在支离破碎中逐步恢复（尽管不均衡），人们将在未来一段时间内承受巨大的痛苦、折磨乃至生活水准下滑。这些问题固然十分关键、痛苦，但它们眼下却不是我关注的重点。我更加关注的是，在地缘政治急剧分裂（早在疫情暴发前就已开始）的背景下，我们的世界正在加速撕裂。我们必须在世界坠下悬崖之前转变方向。新型冠状病毒以及尚在发酵中的气候变化清楚地表明，无论我们愿意与否，我们都身处其中、难以幸免。我们能够超越甩锅游戏和以牙还牙式反应吗？能够避免一个四分五裂的世界在你死我活中坠入深渊吗？或许会更糟？我们能够成为大自然的善良天使吗？能够实现人类的共同命运吗？能够在真正意义上实现全球共同福祉吗？

陌生人的善意

每天，身处封城下的悉尼，在有限的面对面交流中，我都能看到

* 史蒂夫·霍华德，全球基金会秘书长。

人类精神所展现出的积极一面——陌生人的善意。无论是在家里，在
Zoom 上，还是线上音乐会上，人们卸掉了自己的伪装，友善地回应
彼此。我们想让未来变得比现在更好，想把它传承给我们的后代。

好像我们各自社会中的市民精英都渴望加强合作和团结。合作和
团结是地区性的，也是普遍性的。然而，在国际层面和民族国家间依
然会有背道而驰的冲动。地缘政治驶向错误的方向：城堡心态、壁
垒、边界、恐惧和/或仇恨。

新的全球人类安全

教皇方济各曾屡次提及在共同体基础上加强全球人类安全和全球
团结的必要性。我们普遍性的全球目标是，通过对全球共同福祉的向
往，实现真正的人类安全。这将支撑和强化其他所有形式的安全，如
军事安全、经济安全等。然而，在很长时间里，这些安全一直主导和
割裂着国际话语。

民族国家并不是世界唯一的主体。我有个想法：源自我们自身、
内心和群体的路径，而不只是源自政府或其他机构的路径，是否会更
好地通往全球人类安全？姑且称之为自下而上式方法吧，它与自上而
下式方法相对。如果我们每个人都意识到，为了开辟这条路径，进而
实现人类未来在国内、国际上的安全，我们就需要从自身作出一些改
变：心怀谦卑，而非傲慢。

很明显，现有的制度，无论是卫生制度、经济制度还是科技制
度，并未充分地服务社会。哪些问题是紧要的，以及如何在社区、国
家和全球层面有效地就这些问题进行表达和组织，都需要重新进行根
本的评估。换言之，如果需要一场思维和组织的革命，那么这场革命
应该始于我们自己。我从自己的社交网络中感知到了这一点。我觉得
更多的人也感知到了这一点。"我们再也不能像以前那样了。"

西方学习东方

我生活在西方文明中，深受西方文明的影响。我尝试从"他者"

（即来自完全不同的文化背景的那些人）的视角来看待世界，试举一例。众所周知，东亚很多社会的价值体系在很大程度上建立在儒家思想的基础之上。事实上，如果把这些东亚社会加起来，它们将构成世界上最大的经济集团。

整体而言，儒家社会似乎比西方国家受病毒冲击更小。把群体权利置于个人权利之上是儒家的基本要义之一。虽然东亚社会在治理上有些是民主的，有些是集权的（按照我们西方人的说法），但他们在应对病毒方面总体比一些更耀眼的西方国家反应更快，恢复也更好。在这种情况下，谁又能说西方价值和文明更具优越性呢？我们都曾以为，西方思维和制度才是未来全球合作所需要的。

毫无疑问，正如新型冠状病毒所深刻揭示的那样，今后我们应比过去更有效地进行全球合作。

2020 年：重塑全球秩序正当时

自第二次世界大战结束 75 年来，我们一直倚赖的国际秩序被打破了。它需要重建，而不只是修补。2020 年就是一个好的起点，理应让塑造新的全球秩序的声音与其在 21 世纪的相应权重保持一致。

当然，这绝非易事。它困难重重，可能会旷日持久。它需要权力的共享与转移。但如果大国之间无法找到开启对话的合作模式（这似乎是目前的状态），那么中等国家的政府与社会——商业、民间社会、信仰——就得行动起来，努力找到出路。否则，在下一个更致命的病毒出现之前，世界卫生组织和全球卫生合作将会崩塌，世界贸易将在目前停滞的基础上进一步陷入瘫痪，全球气候变化行动将沦为异想天开的托词。世界将进入一个新的"黑暗时期"。

自绝于其他国家和外部世界之外的城堡国家，还将招致更危险的后果。我们曾经看过一部电影，它讲的是此类收缩行为所造成的集聚性影响。它不仅将导致生活质量的下降，还将引发流血冲突。

意愿联盟的重生

我们不妨做个积极的收尾。在各种意愿主体之间，有很多事情要做。我们不妨对"意愿联盟"这一术语进行积极的再利用。这样的联盟可能有很多，也可能混乱不堪、相互重叠，但它们均彰显了人们对无边界思维的渴望。它们应当在"合作性全球化"的精神中绽放，使世界彼此相连、相互依赖。

2013 年，中国在筹建亚洲基础设施投资银行（西方对此反应不一）的过程中，展示了自己的领导意愿，这是国际合作的一个成功范式。此刻，在国家层面、制度层面和经济层面，中国是否愿意在推动完善全球治理模式的对话中发挥领导作用，从而汇聚东西方的国际伙伴？"文明之间的对话"（我喜欢这样的叫法）要求诚实、包容、互鉴和理解，这看似要求很多，但它必将引导我们就国际合作和人类未来存亡的路径问题展开明确、笃实的交流。

让我们携手共创一个变革、公平、包容、繁荣的世界，它将为我们的星球带来最有希望实现的全球人类安全。（王文娥翻译）

原文：

After the Pandemic, What Profound Adjustments Will be Made to the Mode of Collaboration on Pandemic and Climate Change?

Steve Howard[*]

How does this all end? For the moment, as I see it, not that well.

Yes, the world will temper and then eventually overcome the coronavirus. And the global economy will piece itself back together again over time,

---

[*] Steve Howard, Secretary General, Global Foundation.

albeit unevenly, with enormous pain and suffering and lower standards of living for some time to come.

Yet, as critical and painful as these issues are, they are not my main concerns, right now. Our world is fast splintering, in a wild acceleration of the geo-political fracturing we were experiencing before the breakout of the virus.

We need to change direction before the world goes over the cliff. As the virus has so clearly shown and the slower-burning pandemic of climate change is revealing, we are all in this together, whether we like it or not!

Are we capable of rising above blame games and tit for tat responses, of avoiding a descent into hell, of a world divided into blocs, at each other's throats, or worse?

Are we capable of realising the better angels of our nature, of our shared destiny as the human race, of genuinely reaching for the global common good?

The Kindness of Strangers

Every day, I witness this positive side of the human spirit, the kindness of strangers, in my limited face to face contacts in locked-down Sydney. And it's the same at home, in the plethora of Zoom connections and online concerts. People have dropped their pretences and have become themselves. At a deeply personal level, we have faced fear and are responding well. We want to make the future better than the present, to hand on to the next generations.

It's as if the best of civics, as expressed in our respective societies, yearns for stronger co-operation and solidarity, which is local, yes, but at the same time, universal as well.

So why is it that, at the international level, between nation states, there are impulses pulling in the opposite direction? Geo-politics-as expressed by some-is headed the wrong way: fortress mentalities, walls, borders, fear and/or hatred of the other.

Towards a New Global Human Security

Pope Francis has often spoken passionately about the need for stronger global human security, for greater global solidarity, based upon our common humanity. Our universal, global goal might be to achieve true human security through an aspiration for the global common good. This could underpin and trump all other so-called forms of security, such as military and economic, that have for so long dominated and fragmented international discourse.

The nation state is not the only actor in this. Here's an idea: how about a pathway to better global human security that originates not only from governments or other institutions, but from within ourselves, within our own hearts and within our communities? Call it a bottom-up approach, to intersect with top-down. What if we each realised that the changes that may be required to safely navigate a pathway to a secure human future at home and abroad might start within ourselves, with a renewed sense of humility rather than hubris?

It is evident that existing systems, whether of health, markets, technology, have not served society as well as they ought. A more fundamental re-evaluation may be required, about what matters and, in turn, how best that can be expressed and assembled, at community, national and global level. In other words, if a kind of revolution of thinking and organisation is required, it needs to begin within ourselves. I sense this amongst my own networks and I have a hunch that this is felt more widely. "We can't simply go on like before".

The West Learning from the East

As I live in and am a product of Western civilisation, here's an example of my learning to look through the eyes of "the other", those who come from vastly different cultural backgrounds. It is said that the value systems of many societies in East Asia are largely based on Confucian thinking. In fact, I've heard told that, if added together, they would comprise the largest economic bloc in the world!

Broadly, it appears that the largely Confucian societies have been impacted less by the virus than counterparts in the West. A basic tenet of Confucian thinking is to value the rights of the community over the individual. Although these societies are governed across what we in the West would call a democratic-to-authoritarian spectrum, in the main they seem to have pulled together more quickly in their response to the virus and in steps to recovery than some more prominent Western nations.

Who then has the right to that say Western values and civilisation are superior, as we consider the kind of thinking and systems that might be needed for future global co-operation?

Because, make no mistake, as the coronavirus has starkly demonstrated, we are going to need far more effective global co-operation in the future than in the past.

2020 is the Right Time to Reshape Global Arrangements

The international order that served us well for the 75 years since the Second World War, is broken and in·need of re-construction, not just repair. Right now, the 2020 year, is a good place to start, ensuring that the voices in the room that are shaping the new global order are commensurate with their relative weight in this new Century.

This will not be easy. It will be fraught and it may take a while. It requires the sharing and the shifting of power. However, if the biggest powers can't find the *modus operandi* to start the conversation together, which appears to be the case at present, then creative middle powers, from governments and societies-business, civil society, faiths-might have to find a way to get the ball rolling.

Otherwise, the WHO and global health co-operation will sputter until the next, more deadly virus emerges; world trade will further paralyse beyond its stasis today; and global climate change action will remain a rhetorical whimsy. This would truly look like a new Dark Ages.

Heaven knows the even more dangerous consequences that would flow from atomised, fortress states, cut off from each other and the outside world. We've seen this movie before, of the cumulative impact of such reductive actions. It leads not only to a lesser quality of life, it ultimately leads to bloodshed.

Coalitions of the Willing Reborn

Let's conclude on a positive note. There is much to do, between willing actors. Let's re-badge and positively re-use the term, "coalitions of the willing". Such alliances may be multiple, they may be messy and overlapping, all however will involve the need for borderless thinking. They should bloom in the spirit of *"co-operative globalisation"*, that is, for an interconnected and interdependent world.

In 2013, China showed that it was ready to lead-with mixed support from the West, at first—in the formation of the Asian Infrastructure Investment Bank, a successful model of international co-operation. Might it be timely that China, at both State level and also with its think tanks and businesses, could now choose to play a leading role in stimulating dialogues about improved models of global governance, bringing together a variety of international partners, from both East and West?

This "dialogue between civilisations", as I like to call it, will require honesty, tolerance, mutual learning and understanding, a big ask. This, however, is a necessary prelude to the clear-eyed, hard-edged exchanges that should follow, about preferred pathways to international co-operation and human survival in the future.

Let's work together for a world which is transformative, fair, inclusive and prosperous, and which seeks above all else to deliver the best possible global human security on our planet.

新日本在新冠肺炎疫情危机后的政治重组

田中直毅（Naoki Tanaka）*

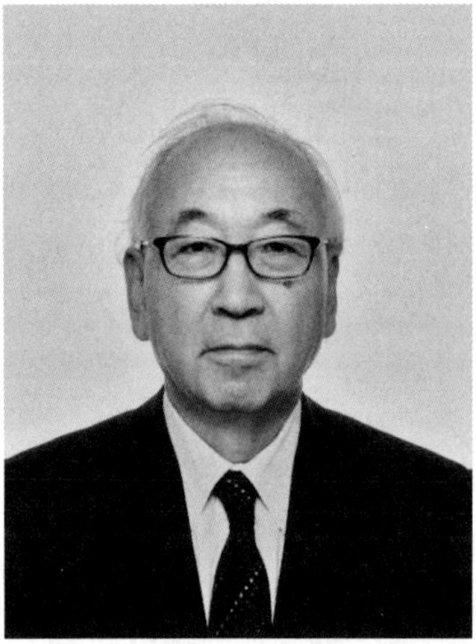

为应对新型冠状病毒大流行，日本式锁城对日本社会产生了许多影响。我们现在发现第二次世界大战之后形成了新的残酷现实。我们社会的自治系统被一一划分，许多孤岛受到它们自己逻辑和实践的支配。新型冠状病毒大流行冲击了我们的社会结构和政治。我现在要举两个在西方民主政治制度下的例子。

联邦德国在第二次世界大战后引入社会市场体系，由市场机制决定资源分配。但为了稳定社会，同时也引入社会干预机制以改善工人的工作环境和生活。当出现严重衰退，企业可以采取及时的裁员措施。当时，通过由雇主和雇员组成的社会保险制度，为下岗工人提供了足够的准备金。为了使社会保险会计制度保持活跃，财政纪律处于和平时期，因为政府预算可能要对社会保险账户进行补助。

在新冠肺炎疫情危机中，德国企业可以迅速采取裁员措施，一旦危机过去，他们就有机会恢复供应系统。因为危机结束后，工人将重

* 田中直毅，日本国际公共政策研究中心理事长。

返工作岗位。当订单量减少时，企业可以降低运营成本。

我们看到德国的财政方面显示出强劲的盈余。他们政治制度的特点就是为这种危机做准备。由于其良好的财政惯例，保证了其社会的可持续性。

以美国为例，他们通过私营企业的竞争发展了市场机制。许多企业努力引入创新实践。政府部门由于依赖私人商业行为而没有扩大操作系统。由于封城，私营部门的现金流受到了严重打击。为了补充私营企业的流动性，应由政府部门吸收有担保的贷款义务和商业票据集体证券。在这种情况下，美国联邦政府将其权力委托给美联储，而美联储选择了 Blacklock（全球最大的资产管理公司）作为代表。在资产管理公司与美联储签订合同之前和之后，都对防火墙原理进行了测试。市场惯例在美国社会中起着非常重要的作用。当和平时期回来后，它们将能够避免大政府的噩梦。

对日本而言，我们的社会既没有像德国这样的社会市场机制框架，也没有像美国那样的深化市场机制的做法。因此，我们的社会冒着大政府的噩梦和巨大的政府部门赤字的风险。在这场危机之后，我们的社会可能会采取改革措施，这对于我们社会的可持续发展将是必要的。

日本社会和政治体系发展不充分的原因是战前的军国主义和战后的驻日盟军总部的占领。但是，在 20 世纪初期，日本内务省希望为我们社会中更为贫困和弱势的阶层提供全面的支持机制。这种哲学尤其存在于该部门的社会部，它们全面考虑了劳动力、住房和社会福利问题。有人说社会部被许多马克思主义者占领，是社会主义的根源。但是，当日本社会走向军国主义时，对日本人民和社会的社会监视成为内务省的主要目标。战争结束后，驻日盟军总部决定将内务省分为三个筒仓。劳动力、住房和社会福利各有各的筒仓。战后，社会市场机制的哲学缺少国家代表。在每个筒仓中，利益集团都有基地。

第二次世界大战后，自由民主党的政权基本继续。他们政权的特点是什么？根据我的理解，所有不同筒仓式决策的集合就是自民党政治的基础。关于安全，《日美安保条约》是我们活动的基础和纲要。

即使在冷战后的安全局势下，加强和扩大条约也是我们社会的主要目标。在国内方面，自民党的政治决策过程存在五个有影响的派阀。农业、公路、邮政、福利和教育等派阀已成为分配财政资源的代表。自1965年发生严重衰退以来，预算赤字持续了55年以上。五个派阀希望成为凯恩斯主义政客。但是，实际上从未提到财政纪律。几年前，累积的国家债务已超过我们GDP的200%。在这些情况下发生了新冠肺炎疫情危机。在封城的第一阶段，农业派阀希望引入肉券，向农民提供补贴。当然，在制定经济补偿措施的最后阶段，这种特定的优惠券计划被取消了。但是，这意味着自民党内部的派阀并没有改变他们的观念。日本社会必须非常深刻地思考我们代表的这种政治行动的后果。

近年来，民粹主义在美国甚至在欧洲，都在迅速发展。但是，通常说日本的政治摆脱了民粹主义。在民粹主义运动中，人们经常说，深层国家扭曲了民主决策过程。政客是通过选举选出的。但是，即使政治体制因选举而改变，未当选的官僚或支持决策的知识分子也起着非常重要的作用。可以说这些方面是民主制扭曲的表现。在美国和欧盟，我们可以区分深层国家。然而，在特朗普和英国脱欧出现之后，政治局势一直在变化。相反，日本的政治制度并未改变。

据我了解，日本最近的政治局势中不存在深层国家。这就是为什么日本民粹主义没有出现的原因。新冠肺炎疫情危机不会立即结束。我们社会的可持续性可能会受到质疑。在这种情况下，我们必须重新定义我们的政治和政治人物的角色。至于政府的行政机构，应该重新考虑其存在的理由。新冠肺炎疫情的受害者一定十分痛苦。但是，通过这些受害者，我们有在我们的社会中拥有可持续基础的政治意愿。政治科学在战后日本的学术界并不流行。现在，日本的社会科学家必须拥有政治学的基础。（杜鹃翻译）

原文:

Political Realignment in Japan after COVID-19 Crisis

Naoki Tanaka *

The coronavirus pandemic and Japanese way of lockdowns have implemented a lots for Japanese civil societies. We are now finding new crude realities which were built after World War Ⅱ. Self-governance systems in our civil societies were divided one by one and a lot of silos were governed by their own logics and practices. The coronavirus pandemic hits our social structures and politics. I am now picking up 2 examples which were introduced under the democratic political systems.

In West Germany, social market systems were introduced after World War Ⅱ. Allocation of resources have been decided by market mechanism. However, in order to stabilize the civil society, social intervention mechanism had been introduced for the improvement of workers' conditions and their lives. When severe recessions come, enterprises can adapt prompt layoffs measures. At that time, enough provisions for laid-off workers are given through social insurance systems which are composed by both employers and employees. In order to keep social insurance accountant system active, fiscal disciplines are being kept in peace time as remedies for social insurance accounts may be required through government budgets.

In COVID-19 crisis, German enterprises could take measures for lay-

---

* Naoki Tanaka, President, Center for International Public Policy Studies, Japan.

offs promptly and they had the opportunity to recover supply systems as soon as the crisis had passed. Because workers would return to their working places after the end of crisis. Enterprises could lower the operating costs when less orders were realized.

When we see the fiscal side of Germany, they show the strong surplus. Characteristics of their political systems are the preparation for this kind of crisis. Because of their sound fiscal practices, they guarantee the sustainability of their civil societies.

In the case of the US, they developed market mechanism through the competitions of private enterprises. A lot of innovative practices were introduced by many enterprises' efforts. And government sectors don't enlarge their operating systems because of their reliance on private business practices. Through their lockdowns, cash flows of private sectors were hit very severely. In order to supplement the liquidities for private businesses, secured loan obligations and collective securities of commercial papers should be absorbed by government sectors. In this case, federal government of US delegate their powers to Federal Reserve Board (FRB) and FRB chose Blacklock which was the biggest asset management company in the world as a representative. Principle of firewall within the asset management company was tested before and after their contracts with FRB. Practices in the market played very important role in the US societies. They would be able to avert big government nightmare when peace time returned.

In the case of Japan, our societies didn't have the framework of social market mechanism like Germany and didn't have the practices of deepening market mechanism like the US. Because of these reasons, our societies have a lot of risks to have big government nightmares and huge deficits of government sectors. After this crisis, our societies might introduce the reformist measures which would be needed for the sustainability of our societies.

The reasons of such insufficient social and political systems in Japan came from militarism in prewar periods and occupation by GHQ after the war. However, at the early of 20th century, Department of Interior in Japan wanted comprehensive support mechanisms for poorer and weaker layers in our society. That kind of philosophy existed especially in Social Division of that Department. Problems of labor, housing and social welfare were considered comprehensively. It was called that Social Division was occupied by a lots of Marxists and it was the sources of socialism. However, when Japan's societies went to militarism, social surveillance of Japanese people and societies became the main objective of the Department of Interior. GHQ after the war decided to divide the Department of Interior into three silos. Labor, housing and social welfare have had each silo. The philosophy of social market mechanism didn't have the state-representative after the war. In each silo, vested interests group had the bases.

After the World War Ⅱ, the regime of Liberal Democratic Party (LDP) continued basically. What were the characteristics of their regime? According to my understanding, collections of every different-silo-type-decision making were the basis of LDP politics. As to the security, Japan-US Security Treaty has been the basis and outlines of our activities. Even in post-cold war security situations, strengthening and expansion of the treaty were the main objectives for our civil society. As to domestic side, five influential tribes existed in LDP political decision making process. Tribes of agriculture, roads, postal services, welfare and education have been representatives for their allocation of fiscal resources. Since 1965 when severe recession took place, deficits of budget continued for more than 55 years. Five tribes wanted to be accepted as Keynesian-type politicians. However, actually in anytime fiscal disciplines were not mentioned. Accumulated national debts became more than 200% of our GDP in several years ago. COVID-19 crisis took place in these situations. At first stage of lockdowns, tribe of agriculture wanted to introduce the coupon of meat to give subsidies to farmers. Of course in the last stage of making the economic compensation measures, such kind of specific coupon scheme was cancelled. However, it meant that tribes within LDP didn't change their mindsets. Japan's societies have to think very deeply the consequence of this kind political actions of our representatives.

In the US, and even in Europe, populism expanded very rapidly in recent years. However, it is usually said that Japan's politics escaped populism. In populistic movement it is said very often that deep states distort democratic decision making processes. Politicians are chosen by elections. However, unelected bureaucrats or decision-support intellectuals play very important role even if political regime changed by elections. It is called that these aspects are representation of distortion of democracies. In the US and EU, we could distinguish deep states. However, after appearance of D. Trump and Brexit, political situations have been changing. On the contrary, Japan's political system didn't change.

According to my understanding, deep states didn't exist in recent political situations in Japan. That's the reason why Japan populism didn't appear.

COVID-19 crisis will not end promptly. Sustainability of our societies might be questioned. In these situations we have to redefine our politics and the role of politicians. As to administration of our government, raison d'etre should be reconsidered.

Victims of COVID-19 must be very unhappy. However, through these victims, we will have the political will to have sustainable basis in our civil societies. Political science was not popular in post war Japan's academic society. Now social scientists in Japan have to have the basis of political science.

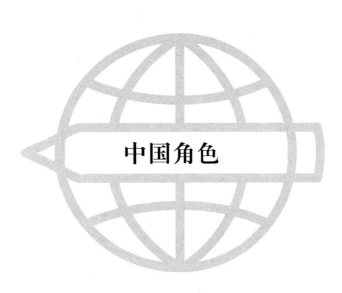

中国角色

中国经济和全球化

——展望未来

彼得·柯西尼（Peter Koenig）[*]

新冠肺炎疫情危机暴发以来，世界也许要经历权力的巨大转变，向更平衡的文明、更强的社会正义和公平转移。为应对新冠病毒肺炎危机，大多数国家政府决定采取封锁措施，世界几乎完全封闭。可能永远无法回到新冠肺炎疫情暴发前的"正常"年代。但这也许不是坏兆头，毕竟在疫情之前，尤其是在西方国家，道德上已经不属于"正常"范畴了。

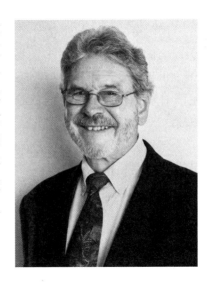

疫情前的全球化与经济发展

新自由主义经济学已经将贪婪、不平等、对人的剥削和资源枯竭"正常化"。这在很大程度上由于越发肆无忌惮的极端资本主义全球化和通过国际合作主义及全球化的私人银行将包括商品、服务和资产在内的一切私有化。

全球金融过去是、某种程度上现在仍然是由法定美元体系主导，

---

[*] 彼得·柯西尼，瑞士经济学家，独立撰稿人，世界银行和世界卫生组织前高级官员。

该体系旨在完全控制全球财富，建立对全球经济和资源的霸权，以制裁和没收资产为手段，并在美国及其西方盟友的支配下胁迫持不同意见的国家。拒绝屈服的国家都遭到了无情的攻击，包括古巴、委内瑞拉、伊朗、叙利亚、也门、朝鲜，当然还有中国和俄罗斯。

新冠肺炎疫情的大蔓延减缓了西方对中国和俄罗斯的施压，造成全球经济活动骤停，引发资产崩溃，导致股市暴跌30%以上，带来史无前例的破产、失业和人类苦难。这场灾难带来的损失可能远远超过1772年的信贷危机、1929—1933年的大萧条和2007—2009年的国际金融危机，甚至可能超出几个数量级。疫情结束后，可以对损失进行更准确的核算。对损失的计算可能耗时几个月，甚至几年。

国际劳工组织初步估计预测，全球约有16亿人失业，约占全球劳动力的一半，其中许多人在疫情暴发前已经生活在不稳定的条件下。世界粮食计划署担心数亿人可能遭受饥荒，数千万人可能因此死亡。让我们在这个暗淡的预测之上，期待并希望迎接一个更光明的未来。

新冠肺炎疫情这朵乌云背后的一丝曙光是美元霸权即将终结，取而代之的是，世界将迎来一扇完全敞开的新机遇之窗，可以打造适合全人类的社会结构，构建新的社会契约，为人类创造共同的未来。

我们了解的全球化显著特征

过去70年里，全球化的资本主义丝毫不受约束，这种模式下发展的经济肆虐发展中国家乃至全球，导致各国民众间和国家间的不平等和不公正急剧增加。《华盛顿共识》（1989年）为缔结不平等的贸易协定提供了可能，而这种协定经常损坏甚至无视较贫穷国家的国家主权，例如，强迫这些国家允许受补贴的农作物进入，导致当地农民不得不离开生活的土壤。

新自由主义理念下的全球化也将一切私有化，尤其是社会服务和基础设施的私有化，摧毁了人们积累的资产基础——将社会资本从底层转移到顶层，转移到西方私人银行和少数寡头手中。这就摧毁了较贫穷国家可能好不容易建立的为数不多且往往脆弱的社会安全网，原本安全网能够在因新冠肺炎疫情造成贫困激增的情况下发挥作用。

中国的毛泽东主席在1949年发起革命，这场革命提出了一个新的经济和社会发展概念，至今仍然有效。在西方对中国施加破坏后，中国非常明智地开始通过在教育、健康和营养方面寻求实现自给自足来增强实力，并消除贫困。中国社会在持续创造的洪流中努力并继续努力，自然，会出现跌宕起伏、不断尝试和发生错误，但中国始终稳步前进、不断学习并取得成功，这反过来又会激发新的创造，也带来新成就。

在实现了基本自主的第一个目标后，中国向世界敞开了大门，继续保持贸易和投资、教育和文化交流方面的和谐关系，并逐步转向研究和尖端科学领域，愿意与世界分享。这与西方的一贯做法相反。中国选择合作而不是竞争。受利润驱动的西方资本主义很难理解这种概念。

经济发展中的合作理念，持续不断的创新，再加上避免冲突、勇往直前的坚定道家原则，中国从70年前的零基础出发，发展到了今天的水平，成为全球第二大经济体。中国是社会主义成功的生动例子。中国是从不寻求冲突或侵略其他国家，而是努力发展伙伴关系并提倡和平共处的国家。这让西方感到担忧，尤其是自命不凡的美帝国。

2013年9月7日，极具远见卓识的习近平主席在哈萨克斯坦的纳扎尔巴耶夫大学重新启动了2100多年前的丝绸之路。为顺应21世纪潮流，倡议名为"一带一路"，但它的基础原则仍然是通过和平、和谐和"双赢"的方式，搭建各国人民之间的桥梁，实现商品、研究、教育、知识、文化智慧之间的交流。

习近平主席在启动仪式上发表了题为《弘扬人民友谊 共创美好未来》的演讲。习近平主席进一步提到了，古丝绸之路上不同信仰和文化民众的交流历史。"交往历史证明，只要坚持团结互信、平等互利、包容互鉴、合作共赢，不同种族、不同信仰、不同文化背景的国家完全可以共享和平，共同发展。"

这是21世纪发展和努力的基石。它标志着不同条件下的全球化——基于平等的全球化。自然，还有新的社会契约。伙伴国家是在邀请下而非胁迫下，参与这项庞大伟业，以陆路和海上路线跨越世界，开展贸易、联合研究和科学交流，为新技术和社会科学带来源源不断的想法，从而推动人类的和平互动。疫情暴发后，中国和古巴在卫生科学领域开展的合作就是一个典型案例。

新常态下的全球化

中国将在新兴世界秩序中发挥重要作用。这种世界秩序不是由西方少数精英所设想而成，不是为了筑墙，而是建立在伙伴关系和平等基础上，以和平和非暴力的方式避免冲突并解决冲突。随之而来的新社会契约能帮助所有有兴趣参与的人了解世界。疫情危机逐渐唤醒人类的新意识，这种新意识是我们一直拥有但却淹没在事物的洪流中——贪婪、权力、舒适以及对弱势和贫困人群的忽视。

中国可能是实现这一新模式的指路明灯。为什么呢？因为在过去70年的革命中，中国已经经历了今天被疫情摧毁的世界所需要的一切。中国重建和重新启动一套新的价值观，在保持环境健康的同时，更好地实现商品、服务和资源获取的平衡。

推动中国向前发展的是一个简单的原则，即通过由主权央行管理的公共银行体系，为当地市场进行本地生产，用当地货币进行本地消费，为人民谋福利（而不是为股东谋私利），努力实现公平发展和所有人的自给自足。丝毫不限制私营部门的参与。但是，国家为出于私人利益的活动制定了规则和参数。因此，中国是"中国特色社会主义国家"。

展望全球化新概念

中国经济很强劲。尽管实际上大概停滞了两个月，但中国经济已基本复苏，而西方国家还在努力寻找合作和经济改革的共同点。国际货币基金组织预测，2020年全球国内生产总值将下降3%，2021年将略有增长。国际货币基金组织预计中国2020年将有1.1%的温和增长量。这两个数字可能都被低估了。鉴于全球经济大规模衰退，2020

年全球国内生产总值（GDP）可能下降高达10%—15%。

另一方面，中国经济已经相当迅速地复苏，公共银行部门必须解决经济的弱点。2020年，中国经济增长率可能在3%—3.5%之间。但正如中国人民大学国际货币研究所（IMI）的首席经济学家所说："我们谈论的是有质量的增长"，这意味着侧重于人们需求的社会层面。

中国将推进"一带一路"倡议这一21世纪的社会经济发展计划，并扩大其倡议的合作伙伴和准成员，目前已有超过160个国家和地区参与。由于疫情灾难，许多国家国内生产总值下降，而外债与之相反不断上升。习近平主席刚刚承诺，中国将投入20亿美元抗击疫情。额外的债务减免，尤其是为债务缠身、较贫穷的"一带一路"倡议参与国减免债务，也许将有助于建设联系更加紧密的世界。

新的全球化将从疫情危机的灰烬中诞生。恢复个别国家的主权，以及它们的货币、金融和经济自主性，同时不让其因债务束缚阻碍自身繁荣发展，这对建立新全球化世界中的平等伙伴关系至关重要。"一带一路"倡议作为一种新工具，可以让有自信的伙伴国不必担心因渴望维护自身主权而受到"制裁"。

西方国家，尤其是美国，可能不喜欢"改变游戏规则"。因此，在可预见的未来，中国可能无法免于西方的抨击和侵略。背后的原因不是美国所谓的疫情内疚或管理不善、贸易不公。这些不实指控意在诋毁中国，希望破坏或削弱世界对中国经济的信任，尤其是对中国由黄金支持的强大货币人民币。

中国人民银行不久前在包括深圳、苏州、成都和雄安在内的多座城市试运行了新推出的加密货币——电子人民币。

终有一日，新的网络货币将在国际上得到推广，用于贸易、大宗商品定价，甚至充当安全稳定的储备货币。数字区块链货币保证了用户的整体安全，不受外界干扰。这是免受"制裁"和随意没收的保护。这也将为中国的经济实力增加一个新维度。中国不仅在经济上将很快超过美国，而且人民币也可能很快成为世界主要储备货币。

广阔的亚欧大陆与非洲相连。为这片巨大的陆地服务，我们无须穿越海洋。贸易简单，关系友好，没有冲突，因为平等的伙伴争取的是真正意义的贸易，没有输家，只有双赢。上海合作组织成员国除中国外，还包括俄罗斯、印度和巴基斯坦等正式成员国，以及伊朗和蒙古国等观察员国。

中国也在促进东盟 10 + 3 国家之间的贸易（东南亚国家联盟包括文莱、柬埔寨、印度尼西亚、老挝、马来西亚、缅甸、菲律宾、新加坡、泰国和越南；" + 3"指中国、韩国和日本）。货币交易将以本币进行，而非美元，交易使用中国人民银行人民币跨境支付系统（CIPS），避免使用由美元控制的 SWIFT 支付系统。

上海合作组织和东盟 10 + 3 的成员国约占世界人口的一半，全球经济产出的三分之一。这是令人生畏的巨大市场，而且大部分国家都在亚欧大陆这片巨大土地上。不需要好战的西方。

这种新形式的非侵略性和非入侵性的全球化可以视作榜样并引起反思。这种全球化也许能够服务于其他国家，比如充当欧洲在严重的新冠肺炎疫情中恢复的工具。让我们畅想一下平等的全球化世界——人类命运共同体。（董方源翻译）

原文：

China's Economy and Globalization

—A Look into the Future

Peter Koenig[*]

After the corona crisis, the world may be facing a monumental para-

---

* Peter Koenig, Economist, Independent writer, Switzerland, Former Senior Official in the World Bank and the World Health Organization.

digm shift of power towards a more balanced civilization—more social justice and equity. The global almost total lockdown, chosen by most governments around the globe in response to mastering the COVID-19 crisis. It may never return to the "normal" of the times before COVID-19. That may not be a bad omen, though, as our pre-corona existence—especially in the west-was everything else but an ethical "normal".

Pre-Corona Globalization and Economic Development

Neoliberal economics have "normalized" greed, inequity, exploitation of people and depletion of resources. This was largely possible due to an ever more reckless ultra-capitalist globalization and privatization of everything-goods, services and assets through international corporatism and globalized private banking.

Global finance was—and still is to some extent—dominated by a fiat US-dollar system aiming at total control of the world's riches towards a global economic and resources hegemony, enforced by sanctions and confiscation of assets, coercing dissenting nations under the dictate of the United States and her western allies. The countries that did not cave in—Cuba, Venezuela, Iran, Syria, Yemen, North Korea-and not least, of course, China and Russia are relentlessly assailed.

The corona pandemic slowed western pressure on China and Russia and brought about an abrupt stop to world economic activities, causing a meltdown of assets, plunging stock markets by over 30 percent, creating untold bankruptcies, unemployment and human misery unrecorded in past history. The calamity may be far surpassing the Credit Crisis of 1772, the Great Depression (1929 – 1933) and the Financial Crisis of 2007 – 2009, possibly by orders of magnitude, once the dust settles and a more accurate accounting can take place. This may take months, if not years.

First estimates from the International Labor Office (ILO) predict unemployment to reach about 1. 6 billion people, worldwide, about half the globes workforce, many of them living in precarious conditions well before the corona outbreak. The World Food Program (WFP) fears that hundreds of millions of people may be affected by famine and tens of millions may die. This is a somber base from which to look forward into—let's hope—a brighter future.

The silver lining of this dark corona cloud is that the dollar hegemony is coming to an end, and instead the world is presented with a wide-open window of new opportunities to stitch a social fabric that fits all of humanity— forging a new social contract towards creating a common future for mankind.

Salient Features Under Globalization as We Know It

Economic development under unfettered globalized capitalism has in the past 70 years ravaged the globe and in the Global South has drastically increased inequality, injustice among peoples and nations. The Washington Consensus (1989) has given free reign for forging unequitable trade agreements which often undermined and even annihilated national sovereignties of poorer countries, for example, driving local farmers off their land by forcing subsidized agricultural crops into their countries.

Globalization under the neoliberal concept has also brought privatization of everything, but especially of social services and infrastructure, destroying the peoples' accumulated asset base-shuffling social capital from the bottom to the top, to the western private banking sector and a few oligarchs, thereby destroying the little and often flimsy social safety nets poorer nations may have established—safety nets which would come in handy now with COVID – 19 caused poverty skyrocketing.

China's 1949 Revolution initiated by Chairman Mao presented a new concept of economic and social development, one that still holds as of today. After western devastation of China, it started wisely in building strength by seeking self-sufficiency in education, health and nutrition-and in eradicating poverty. The Chinese society worked and keeps working in a flux of constant creation—with natural ups and downs and trials and errors—but steadily advancing, learning-and succeeding which, in turn, motivates new creation, new achievements.

After reaching this first objective of basic autonomy, China opened her gates to the world to continue the harmonious flow of creating relationships for trade and investments, educational and cultural exchange and gradually moving into research and cutting-edge science to share with the world. It is the contrary of what the west is used to. It is cooperation instead of competition. A concept hardly understood in the profit-driven capitalist west.

The idea of cooperation in economic development coupled with an endless flow of creation-avoiding conflicts and moving forward, a solid Tao principle-has grown China to where she stands today-becoming the world's second largest economy, after starting practically from zero only 70 years ago. China is a vivid example of socialist success. A nation that never seeks conflicts or invasions of other countries, but strives for partnerships and peaceful cohabitation. This worries the west, especially the self-declared US empire.

On 7 September 2013, Visionary President Xi Jinping re-initiated the ancient 2100-year-old Silk Road at Kazakhstan's Nazarbayev University. Adjusted to the 21st Century, it is called the Belt and Road Initiative (BRI), but it is based on the same old principles building bridges between-peoples, exchanging goods, research, education, knowledge, cultural wisdom, peacefully, harmoniously and 'win-win' style.

In his inauguration speech, President Xi spoke about "Promote Friendship Between Our People and Work Together to Build a Bright Future". But he went further, pointing to the history of exchanges under the Ancient Silk Road among people from different creeds and cultures, "they had proven that countries with differences in race, belief and cultural background can absolutely share peace and development as long as they persist in unity and mutual trust, equality and mutual benefit, mutual tolerance and learning from each other, as well as cooperation and win-win outcomes. "

This is the cornerstone for the development endeavor of the 21st century. It signals a globalization under different terms-a globalization under equals. And, yes, a New Social Contract. Partner countries are invited, not coerced, to participate in this mammoth enterprise to span the world with land and maritime routes, for trade, for joint research and scientific exchanges, leading to an endless flow of ideas for new technologies but also of social sciences to enhance peaceful human interactions. A case in point may be the new China-Cuba collaboration in health science that emerged from the corona crisis.

Globalization Under a New Normal

China will play a major role in the new emerging world order—not a One World Order, as a small Western elite envisions, but a new paradigm built on partnership, on equality on building bridges, instead of walls, avoiding and resolving conflicts peacefully and without violence. Call it a new Social Contract to span the world for all those who are interested in participating. The COVID-19 pandemic is gradually bringing an awakening for a new consciousness, one that we always had but got buried in the rush of things-greed, power, comfort and also neglect for the less privileged and destitute.

China may be a guiding light for the realization of this new paradigm. Why? Because China experienced in her 70 years of Revolution what the corona-devastated world needs today to rebuild and to restart with a new set of values towards a better equilibrium of access to goods, services and resources, while maintaining a healthy environment.

What propelled China forward, was the simple principle of local production for local markets and local consumption with a local currency through a public banking system managed by a sovereign central bank working for the good of the people (not for shareholders), gearing towards an equitable development and self-sufficiency for all. This does not preclude private sector participation at all. But the State sets rules and parameters within which private interests may move. That's why China is "A socialist nation with Chinese characteristics."

Prospects for a New Concept of Globalization

China's economy is strong. Despite a practical standstill of about two months, China has almost recovered, while the west is still struggling to find common denominators for collaboration and for revamping their economies. The IMF has predicted a global GDP decline of 3% for 2020, and a slight growth for 2021. For China the IMF foresees a modest growth of 1.1% in 2020. Both figures are likely underestimated. Given the massive wipe-out of much of the global economy, 2020 negative GDP for the world may be as high as 10% to 15% when the chips are down and counted.

On the other hand, China having recovered rather quickly and with a public banking sector destined to address the economy's weak spots, 2020 growth might be in the order of 3% to 3.5%. But as a leading economist from the International Monetary Institute (IMI) of Beijing's Renming University says— "we are talking about quality growth", meaning it will focus on the social dimension of people's needs.

China will forge ahead with the socioeconomic development program of the century-the BRI and expand her partner and associate members, already more than 160 today. Due to the corona catastrophe, foreign debt has been rising almost in reverse proportion as GDP has declined. President Xi has just pledged 2 billion dollars to fight the virus. Additional debt relief especially to the poorer debt-strangled Belt and Road partners, might facilitate progress towards a better-connected world.

A new kind of globalization will emerge from the ashes of the corona crisis. Restoring individual countries sovereignty, as well as their monetary, financial and economic autonomy and without a debt stranglehold preventing them from prospering, is crucial for becoming equal partners in a new globalized world. BRI is the new vehicle promoting self-assured partners that do not have to fear "sanctions" for wanting to preserve their sovereignty.

The west, especially Washington may not like this "game changer" approach. Therefore, China may not be spared in the foreseeable future from western bashing and aggressions. The reasons are NOT corona guilt or mismanagement, or unfair trade, reasons Washington likes to propagandize. These false accusations are meant to denigrate China to break or weaken the world's trust in China's economy and in particular her strong and gold backed currency, the yuan.

People's Bank of China, PBC has just launched a trial run in a number of cities, including Shenzhen, Suzhou, Chengdu, and Xiong'an of her new crypto-currency, the e-RMB (Ren Min Bi, meaning People's Money), or Yuan.

Eventually the new cyber money will be rolled out internationally for trade, commodity pricing—and even as a safe and stable reserve currency. The digital blockchain money assures the users total security, no interference from outside. It is a protection from "sanctions" and arbitrary confiscation. This will add a new dimension to China's economic strength. Not only will her economy soon outrank that of the United States, but the yuan may also shortly become the key reserve currency in the world.

Look at the huge continent of Eurasia which is also connected to Africa. To serve this enormous landmass no seas have to be crossed. Its easy trading, friendly relations, no conflicts, because equal partners strive for the real meaning of trade, no losers, only win-win. Then there are the countries of the Shanghai Cooperation Organization (SCO), which in addition to China include also Russia, India and Pakistan—and soon also Iran, with Malaysia and Mongolia in observation status waiting in the wings.

China is also boosting trade among the ASEAN +3 countries (Association of Southeast Asian Nations: Brunei, Cambodia, Indonesia, Laos, Malaysia, Myanmar, the Philippines, Singapore, Thailand, and Vietnam; plus 3 means Japan, South Korea and China). Monetary transactions will take place in local currencies, not the US dollar. They will be using CIPS (Cross-Border Interbank Payment System), avoiding the dollar controlled SWIFT payment scheme.

SCO and ASEAN + 3 account for about half the world population and for one third of the globes economic output. It is a formidable market and most of it on this huge landmass called Eurasia. No need for the belligerent west.

This new form of non-aggressive and non-invasive globalization may make example and evoke reflection. Perhaps it may serve others, Europe for instance—as a vehicle to recover from the colossal corona collapse. Imagine a globalized world among equals—a community seeking a common future for mankind.

新冠肺炎疫情：世界危机的催化剂及中国的新角色

拉丁美洲社会科学理事会
"中国与世界权力版图"研究小组

新冠肺炎疫情暴发后，引发了一场其对全球权力版图影响的大讨论。21世纪以来，全球权力版图不断经历着变化，尤其是2008年的国际金融危机，深刻改变了世界格局。时至今日，全球尚未完全走出那场经济危机带来的重创，2020年1月起又陷入了新冠肺炎疫情引发的危机。毋庸置疑，这场疫情成了世界格局调整的催化剂或加速器。

全球地缘政治新格局？

新冠肺炎疫情会带来哪些综合影响？面对疫情采取的不同应对措施对资本主义的运行和全球权力版图会产生何种影响？在现阶段，这些影响尚无法清晰、准确地显现。我们身处的时代充满各种不确定性。新冠病毒肺炎恰如一张"变牌"，它的出现至少让我们确定了一件事：世界已然改变，那个我们在2019年12月告别的世界已不复存在。

一系列变化随之而来，如全球地缘政治新格局的形成、对新自由主义全球化的质疑、技术范式的转变等。与此同时，一种新的积累模式在全球范围内引发普遍关注。这种新的积累模式基于快速发展的技术变革以及不同于西方社会工程学的一种全新的"公民—政府—市场"关系构建而成。该积累模式的标杆主要是在亚洲，中国最为典型。鉴于此，可以预见，老牌发达国家与正在崛起的大国在拉丁美洲和加勒比地区的地缘政治角力将进一步加剧。

在中美贸易摩擦（其背景是一场科技竞争和地缘经济竞争）取得脆弱的休战后，中美之间的地缘政治竞争在疫情期间日益加剧，尤其是在舆论领域，如声称中国应对席卷全球的新冠肺炎疫情负责，将新冠肺炎疫情视为中国作为强国的终结等。但短短几日，现实就有力驳斥了西方的上述言论。中国积极开展国际合作，在全球抗疫中扮演了重要角色（当然，还有俄罗斯和古巴）。

与此形成鲜明对比的是，美国和欧盟的表现令人十分失望。欧盟成立的初衷面临轰塌。欧盟先是没有出台任何统一措施应对疫情，而后姗姗来迟的道歉亦无法挽救其岌岌可危的形象。在欧盟最需要采取联合行动、统一协作的时刻，成员国之间的合作却偏偏缺席了。

面对新冠肺炎疫情在国内的蔓延，美国政府不负责任的反应有损其政府形象。但秉持民族主义和反全球化的美国政府仍一意孤行，采取更为激进的行动，频频抨击数家多边组织。这些组织机构系美国在第二次世界大战后推动成立，是其霸权体系的组成部分。新近受到抨击的就是世界卫生组织。

新冠肺炎疫情加速巩固了中国在世界舞台上的地位。早在2001年，美国就已将中国这个亚洲巨人视为战略竞争对手，在发展合作关系的同时又采取了一系列措施遏制中国。此后，随着2008—2009年形成的金砖国家合作机制的不断发展，中国逐渐减少购买美国国债，并在全球范围启动企业收购。中国更是于2013年发起"一带一路"倡议。上述种种都是重构世界体系之争中的一部分，中国与美帝国主义的关系进一步恶化，这场全球竞争更趋混杂和碎片化，地缘政治争端也随之加剧。

去全球化、第四次工业革命及中国提供的新积累模式

预测认为，新冠肺炎疫情过后，最保守意义上的民族主义将会反弹。当然，这一趋势早在疫情暴发前就已显露征兆。新自由主义全球

化的主要指标在多年前就开始呈现颓势。就此而言，2008—2010 年的危机构成了转折点。此后，国际贸易、外国直接投资等开始放缓，至今尚未恢复活力。

通过比较应对新冠肺炎疫情措施的有效性，亚洲国家，特别是中国，引领并有效执行的生物技术新范式发挥了积极作用，取得的成效有目共睹。此外，不论是政府组织能力、清理消毒技术，还是公共卫生领域，中国等亚洲国家都更胜一筹（韩国和越南也证明了这一点）。相反，大部分西方发达国家在应对疫情挑战时的无能则一览无遗。

中国对市场社会主义进行了更高层次的变革，正以超出他们预期的发展速度进一步推进经济建设，展示了他们对市场社会主义的改革是行之有效的。中国已具备足够的物质条件以保障其能够几乎毫无障碍地去发展经济。中国经济体制的运行几乎不受金融、外部条件和产能等瓶颈的束缚。中国先进的人机工程学和社会工程学正是在此基础上构建而成的，其优越性已在这场抗疫之战中得到了检验。与此同时，这种经济体制也构成了经济过度金融化的对立面。如今，过度金融化无疑加剧了西方道德危机和智力的衰退。

需要强调的是，2008 年经济危机后，西方国家采取了紧缩政策。而当下，正是那些紧缩政策以及限制公共支出政策对西方自由主义政府（除德国等几个国家外）造成了重重阻碍，使它们无法体面地应对危机。不同于西方国家，中国并未实施紧缩政策。此外，中国在解决市场经济和社会主义这对经典逻辑困境方面也取得了进步。诚然，环境、社会、政治等问题在中国仍然存在，但与此同时，中国出台了一系列解决上述问题的政策，如让内需成为经济发展主引擎、外国直接投资的规范化，以及不局限于一般的道路模式，而是着眼于中国特色社会主义建设等。

一方面，倡导加强欧美合作的人和推崇全球主义的人之间的矛盾日益凸显；另一方面，中国则积极"连接"多极化，以引领世界格局。面对疫情的全球大暴发，中国积极提供国际援助并进一步推动基础设施建设，而后者正是"一带一路"最鲜明的特点。中国的这些项目甚至在欧洲也取得了进展。

新冠肺炎疫情引发的危机表明，有必要"摆脱"新自由主义全球化以应对全球疫情的挑战，至少应迅速反应。多年来，中国一直在设计自己的发展模型。当然，中国并无意说服其他国家接受其发展模型的普遍性。不论考虑采用何种发展模式，一定要深思熟虑，先想清楚哪些可以交由市场，哪些却不能。显而易见，像卫生、教育和某些特定经济部门就不能交由"无形的手"，否则，在中期就会付出昂贵的经济、社会和人力代价。这就是新冠肺炎疫情留给我们的惨痛教训。近几十年来，世界上大部分国家都采用了新自由主义模式，但这次疫情无疑对这一模式产生了巨大冲击。

众所周知，全球化进程陷入停滞，资本角逐加剧危机，两者相互关联，相互影响，并由此引发了一系列矛盾、困境与挑战。如外围经济结构有可能因过度金融化或过于依赖北半球经济而遭受损失；劳资关系进一步紧张；许多国家试图恢复其某些领域的工业化生产，这必将在全球激化更多的矛盾；之前的价值创造模式已经过时（由此造成了对价值的巨大破坏），并出现了新的价值创造模式。与此同时，第四次工业革命使半外围国家陷入了"加入"或者"绝对外围"的困境，并且还有可能使反霸权势力重新出现。

世界权力及其在拉美的新版图

今天的中国已成为拉丁美洲甚至是全球的榜样。通过地缘政治合作，中国已获得了世界引领者的地位，并时刻准备承担起构建其领导地位所需要的经济成本。中国基于内需构建的新发展模式，必将对非洲和拉丁美洲的经济产生影响。随着西方自由主义民主模式及其在外围施加/强加的既定发展模式的危机进一步加剧，一幅全新的矛盾冲突图已然形成。

疫情当前，拉美地区正在经历新旧危机的双重打击，但与此同时，拉美应该利用这一时机重新思考、适时调整一系列政策，如农业生产，特别是农业出口、卫生和教育援助、提高产能及产业结构多样化、推动一体化进程等。

对拉美而言，危机亦是机遇。而这一机遇要求拉美认真规划，制定对华战略政策，而非任其自然发展。风险在于，在全球危机下，榨取性的原材料出口或将进一步加剧，而拉美国内市场的产业结构多样化改革却可能停滞不前。

拉美是一个由多个独立自主的国家组成的地区，亟须重申这一观点并应基于此去思考拉丁美洲。此外，还应时刻秉持拉丁美洲的批判性思维。最后，拉美亟须摒弃欧美的殖民视角，构建一种"立足于我们的拉美看中国"的视角。（楼宇翻译）

原文：

COVID-19：Catalizador de la Crisis Mundial y el nuevo Papel de China

Grupo de Trabajo CLACSO China y el mapa de podermundial

El surgimiento del nuevo coronavirus/COVID-19 ha estimulado el debate sobre su impacto en el mapa de poder mundial que se viene configurando desde principios del siglo XXI. Esta reconfiguración de la geografía del poder tiene lugar en el marco de la crisis global que azota al sistema desde el 2008; y desde enero de 2020 a la crisis global en marcha, se suma la pandemia, la que algunos teóricos del sistema han pretendido presentar como causa de la crisis, cuando realmente ha sido un fatídico catalizador o acelerador de procesos en desarrollo.

¿Una nueva geopolítica global?

Los efectos que tendrán en el funcionamiento del capitalismo y en el mapa de poder global la conjunción de la crisis y las respuestas diferenciadas en el enfrentamiento a la pandemia no pueden ser visualizados con precisión en este momento. Es un momento de incertidumbres, pero la COVID-19, que apareció en el escenario como una wild card, nos deja una certeza: el mundo no será igual al quedespedimos en diciembre de 2019.

Los cambios que se avecinan tienen que ver con un nuevo orden geopolítico, el cuestionamiento a la globalización neoliberal, el cambio del paradigma tecnológico y la visibilización global de un nuevo patrón de acumulación cuyo referente estará en Asia, especialmente en China, asentado en la aceleración del cambio tecnológico y una relación ciudadano-Estado-mercado basada en una nueva ingeniería social distinta a la de Occidente. En este nuevo contexto es previsible la profundización de la disputa geopolítica sobre América Latina y el Caribe entre los poderes globales establecidos y emergentes.

Luego de un débil armisticio en la guerra comercial, la cual expresa de fondo una guerra tecnológica y geoeconómica, el terreno de la disputa geopolítica entre China y Estados Unidos se acrecienta en plena pandemia en el plano retórico, como parte de la guerra por la legitimidad: al de acusar a China como responsable de la pandemia (virus chino) y atribuir a ésta el fin de China como potencia (Chernobyl chino). Bastaron pocos días para que la realidad se encargara de refutar la premonición de Occidente: China se erige en el gran actor de la cooperación internacional, acompañada por Rusia y Cuba.

En contraste, la gran decepción la han protagonizado Estados Unidos y la Unión Europea. La auto narrativa de esta última se desplomó, no ha habido siquiera un protocolo común para enfrentar la pandemia y las tardías disculpas del organismo no serán suficientes para rescatar la imagen de un proyecto en crisis. Cuando más necesaria era su acción conjunta la cooperación estuvo ausente.

Al gobierno nacionalista y anti-globalista de Estados Unidos no le bastó con el descrédito ocasionado por la irresponsable respuesta gubernamental frente al avance de la pandemia en su país, sino que profundizaron su accionar y arremete contra las instituciones multilaterales cuya creación impulsó después de la Segunda Guerra Mundial como parte de su arquitectura hegemónica. La última en sufrirlo fue la OMS.

La pandemia acelera la consolidación del papel de China como actor global, pero es un proceso que también venía de antes, porque desde 2001 Estados Unidos ya había reconocido el gigante asiático como un competidor estratégico y planteaba relaciones de cooperación que a la vez buscaban la contención. Entre 2008 y 2009 se produjo el lanzamiento de los BRICS, acompañado de una cierta institucionalización, y China redujo la compra de bonos del Tesoro de Estados Unidos, así como activó la adquisición de empresas globales y lanzó, en 2013, la Iniciativa de la Ruta y la Franja (BRI), considerada una respuesta al impulso del TPP por las fuerzas globalistas. Estos movimientos son parte de la lucha por la reconfiguración del Orden Mundial que exacerban las reacciones imperiales de Estados Unidos y alimentan la guerra mundial híbrida yfragmentada y la disputa geopolítica.

Desglobalización, Cuarta Revolución Industrial y el nuevo padrón chino de acumulación

Los pronósticos del mundo post-pandemia apuntan a un repunte del nacionalismo en su versión más conservadora, sin embargo, señales de este proceso se registraron con anterioridad. Desde hace varios años se vienen observando retrocesos en los principales indicadores de la globalización neoliberal, en este sentido la crisis de 2008 – 2010 marcó un punto de inflexión tras el cual no ha habido recuperación del dinamismo en el comportamiento del comercio, la IED, etc.

Al mismo tiempo, la efectividad comparada en el combate a la COVID-19 ha evidenciado el papel que en ello ha jugado un nuevo paradigma biotecnológico liderado y gestionado de manera fluida por los países asiáticos, especialmente por China. Junto a la capacidad para articular Estado, tecnologías limpias y salud pública (como también se demostró en el caso de Corea del Sur y Vietnam), la mayor parte de los países desarrollados de Occidente han dado muestras de su incapacidad para enfrentar este desafío. China está validando un cambio de nivel superior del socialismo de mercado, avanzando en la construcción de una economía con una capacidad superior de proyección de su desarrollo. Para ello ha desarrollado condiciones materiales que le permiten operar con restricciones casi cero. Esto significa que es una nueva variante de planificación que trabaja casi sin estrangulamientos (financieros, externos, capacidad productiva instalada, etc.). Esa es la base que sustenta la avanzada ingeniería humana y social cuya fortaleza se puso a prueba en el combate a la pandemia. Y es la antítesis de la financiarización que acelera la decadencia moral e intelectual que hoy afecta a Occidente.

Es importante subrayar que, a diferencia de Occidente tras la crisis de 2008, China no implementó políticas de austeridad y hoy son esas políticas las que impiden a los gobiernos liberales occidentales enfrentar de una manera decorosa la crisis, con sus restricciones del gasto público (salvo excepciones como Alemania y algunos más). Y ha avanzado en dar respuesta al clásico dilema entre economía de mercado y socialismo. Es una sociedad no exenta de contradicciones, en la que persisten problemas medio ambientales, sociales y políticos, pero existen políticas encaminadas a resolverlos, en especial, la conversión del mercado interno en el principal motor de la economía, la regulación de la IED y una perspectiva no enmarcada en un modelo general, sino la construcción del socialismo con características chinas.

Las contradicciones entre los "decadentes" proyectos continentalistas europeo y estadounidense y las fuerzas globalistas se hacen visibles, al tiempo que China asume el liderazgo como articuladora del multipolarismo, ofreciendo ayuda internacional frente a la pandemia eimpulsando obras de infraestructura, que tienen en el BRI su expresión concreta más visible, con avances incluso en Europa.

El impacto de la pandemia ha demostrado la necesidad de "salirse" de la globalización neoliberal para responder a los desafíos de la pandemia, por lo menos como reacción inmediata. China no tiene pretensiones de convencer al resto del mundo de la universalidad de su modelo de desarrollo, durante años trabajó para diseñar un modelo propio. Al pensar cualquier modelo de desarrollo es vital preguntarse qué cosas pueden dejarse al mercado y que no, obviamente la salud, la educación y determinados sectores económicos no pueden dejarse al gobierno de la mano invisible sin pagar altísimos costos económicos, sociales y humanos en el mediano plazo. Es una triste lección que deja la COVID-19, lo cual golpea al modelo neoliberal dominante en gran parte del mundo en las últimas décadas.

El estancamiento de la globalización tal y como la hemos conocido, la aceleración de la crisis estimulada por la lucha entre los capitales, son procesos interrelacionados que abren un abanico de contradicciones, dilemas y desafíos, como la posibilidad de pérdida de las estructuras económicas en la periferia si se quedan atadas a la financiarización y al Norte Global; la agudización de las tensiones capital-trabajo; la tentativa de muchos sectores de las potencias atrasadas de intentar recuperar sus producciones industriales, generando más contradicciones en la economía mundial; la obsolescencia de las formas anteriores de generación del valor (por lo tanto, produce una enorme destrucción de valor) y surgimiento de nuevas formas económicas organizativas de funcionamiento de los procesos de creación de valor. Al mismo tiempo, la 4a Revolución Industrial plantea la disyuntiva de incorporarse o de la "periferización absoluta" para las semiperiferias, y crea también la posibilidad de reemergencia de fuerzas anti hegemónicas.

El nuevo mapa del poder mundial y la América Latina

China ha pasado hoy a ser un país de referencia para la región y el mundo, dispuesta a asumir los costos económicos de la construcción de su liderazgo y ha hecho uso geopolítico de la cooperación como vía para lograrlo. Sin embargo, la asunción de un nuevo modelo de desarrollo por parte de China, basado en la demanda interna, tendrá impactos en las economías africanas y latinoamericanas. En la medida que se aceleran la crisis tanto del modelo de democracia liberal occidental como de los modelos de desarrollo establecidos/impuestos a la periferia, se conforma un nuevo mapa de contradicciones. Si bien es un momento crítico para la región, en que se unen los

efectos de la crisis y los de la pandemia, también es un momento de oportu-
nidades emanadas de replantear/rectificar/cómo se enfrentan: la producción
agrícola, en especial la exportadora; la asistencia a la salud y a la
educación; elaumento de la complejidad productiva; o la integración.

Para la región, la crisis es un momento de oportunidad y ese momento
exige un plan, una estrategia para la relación con China, no se puede dejar
a la espontaneidad que implica reproducir relaciones de dependencia. El pel-
igro es reforzar economías extractivistas primario exportadoras, en crisis
mundial, sin complejidad productiva en el mercado interno y sin control/
democratización de los excedentes producidos en las actividades extracti-
vas. Pensar la región con autonomía y respaldo en el pensamiento crítico lati-
noamericano es una necesidad impostergable. Y también lo es construir una
mirada de China desde Nuestra América, más allá de las anteojeras coloni-
ales.

学习借鉴中国脱贫经验

扎伊迪·萨塔尔（Zaidi Sattar）[*]

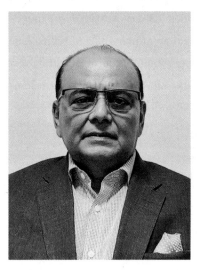

2015 年，联合国大会通过了到 2030 年消除贫困的可持续发展目标（SDG）。该目标呼吁各国采取行动，以消除贫困，保护地球，确保所有人都能共享和平与繁荣。联合国大会通过的这 17 项可持续发展目标不仅包含消除贫困的内容，还呼吁各国制定出台有效的政策，以包容的方式创造财富，同时可持续地利用地球丰富的自然资源，进而做出全面的努力，改善全人类的生存状况。因此，财富的创造和分配也是该目标的重要内容。

如今，贫困现象随处可见，在全球范围内消除贫困的呼声和需求也愈加强烈。同时，消除贫困之路充满了各种艰巨的挑战。所以，虽然人们对这项计划的可行性心存怀疑，但这项跨度长达 15 年的目标路线图仍意义深远。这项计划的可行性到底如何？历史经验和跨国证据为那些拥有大量贫困人口、脱贫资源极其有限的国家，特别是亚非拉的发展中国家提供了一些有益的经验。而中国的减贫经验能为这些国家提供有意义的战略指导。

虽然这次新冠肺炎疫情为全球的脱贫任务增添了新的挑战，但中国 30 年的减贫经验仍能为发展中国家提供借鉴。拥有 14 亿人口的中

* 扎伊迪·萨塔尔，孟加拉国政策研究中心主席。

国是世界上人口最多的国家，而现在只有不到一千万的人被认为是
"极度贫困"。依据世界银行的标准，每日收入低于1.9美元被视为
"极度贫困"。2015年，中国的极度贫困人口占总人口的0.7%，而
这一比例在1981年高达53%。在此期间，中国依靠高效的发展战略，
使约6亿人摆脱了贫困。对于如此庞大的人口基数而言，这样的脱贫
速度在历史上绝无仅有。

在这过去的几十年间，全球各国在减贫方面取得了显著进展。
根据最新的统计，现在全球9%的人口生活在每天1.9美元的极度
贫困线下，而在1990年极度贫困人口比例将近36%。但是今天，
全球仍有7.8亿人生活在贫困中，超过了中国总人口的一半，这一
数字高得令人难以接受，说明经济发展所带来的红利并未在各地区
和国家间均衡分配。亚太国家在消除贫困方面最为成功，其次是南
亚和拉美。但是，撒哈拉以南非洲国家仍顽固地拒绝采取措施进行
减贫（见表1）。

表1　　　　　　　　　1990—2015年各地区极度贫困率情况

地区	贫困率（%），1990年	贫困率（%），2015年
亚太	61.5	2.3
南亚	47.3	12.4
拉美	14.2	4.1
撒哈拉以南非洲	54.3	41.1
全球	35.9	8.6*
中国	53.0**	0.7

资料来源：世界银行；（＊）为2018年数据，（＊＊）为1981年数据。

不管发生在何处，贫困都像是一个诅咒。全世界的穷人都生活
在肮脏的环境中，缺少基本的生活必需品，如充足的食物、住房、
教育和医保等。这些东西在一般人看来司空见惯。21世纪，科技跨
越国界，取得了迅猛发展。与此同时，全球每十个人中就有一人
（近8亿人）生活在贫困之中。这一事实给人类文明在过去几个世
纪取得的所有成就蒙上了一层阴影。国家和全球所面临的这些重要
挑战阻碍了社会进步，使得大批人生活在贫困中。经济增速放缓、

宏观经济失衡、贸易紧张局势升级、收入和机会不均、气候变化、国际关系日益脆弱，冲突加剧，这些因素进一步阻碍了减贫工作和包容性增长。

因此，国际社会应当最终认识到采取行动的时机已经到来。但从目前来看，全球范围内消除贫困的工作进展并不平衡，同时也缺少到2030年实现极度贫困清零目标所必需的条件和资源。根据最新的预测，这一目标可能无法按期实现。联合国2019年度可持续发展目标进度报告发现，生活在极度贫困中的人口比例从1990年的36%下降至2018年的8.6%。但是，随着全球各国疲于应付深度贫困、暴力冲突和自然灾害，减贫工作的步伐开始放缓。此外，全球饥饿指数在保持长期下降态势后最近又有所回升。现在，新冠肺炎疫情又加剧了这些挑战，疫情阻断了全球的经济活动，对许多国家和地区的就业、收入和粮食产出造成了巨大的负面冲击。疫情可能会使减贫日程表倒退几年。此次疫情在卫生和经济领域造成了前所未有的冲击。我认为，将可持续发展目标的期限调整到2035年是一种切实可行的做法。

那么，一项成功的、能有效消除贫困的发展战略应包括哪些关键因素？在高速发展、创造就业和减贫方面，发展中国家可以从中国学习借鉴到哪些经验？

1979年，中国开始从计划经济向市场经济过渡。当时，中国是一个贫穷的、内向型的国家，人均国民收入182美元，贸易依存度（贸易额与国内生产总值之比）为11.2%。自那以后，中国在经济领域的表现堪称奇迹。1980—2010年的30年间，中国的国内生产总值保持了年均10%的增长，国际贸易年均增长16%。现在，中国已经是中等偏上收入国家，6亿多人口成功脱贫。贸易依存度达到65%，位居世界主要经济体之首。2009年，中国超过日本成为世界第二大经济体，同年取代德国成为世界最大商品出口国。中国常被委婉地称为"世界工厂"。是什么样的发展战略使得中国取得了这些成绩？

将中国所取得的成就总结为某种战略未免过于简单草率了。但在诸多因素中，中国采取的对外开放和贸易导向政策无疑发挥了关键作用。20世纪六七十年代，亚太地区出现了一种新的发展模式，即贸易主导型发展模式。当时，"东亚四小龙"作为典范，利用巨大的全球市场，获得了快速发展。同时，全球巨大的需求量也为"东亚四小龙"的商品提供了一个深度、弹性的市场。1979年，中国采取了改革开放政策，较之"东亚四小龙"又向前迈进了一步。中国很快意识到，国际贸易和知识转移是实现快速发展的重要战略来源。通过向国际市场开放贸易活动，中国在全球范围内为其制造的产品开拓了巨大的需求，同时还引进了有助于提高生产效率的知识。

同样重要的是，中国遵循了正确的工业化顺序：首先，与许多发展中国家推行的比较优势违背（CAD）进口替代战略不同，中国的出口和工业扩张是建立在其庞大的廉价劳动力基础上的，这是一种比较优势遵循（CAF）战略。其次，通过从世界各地引进思想、技术和技巧，中国得以运用更先进的技术。总之，中国引进了世界的知识，输出了世界的需求。同时，来自世界的需求为中国的工业带来了国内市场所欠缺的规模经济。

中国所采取的另一项战略是谋求结构变革，包括工业化、城镇化和创造就业机会。历史上看，世界上所有国家在现代化之初都是贫穷的农业国家。而其中，只有少数国家转贫为富。这些国家无一例外都采取变革，将农村农业经济转变为城市工业经济。中国也效仿了以上做法，但稍有不同。当失业的人们从农村地区来到城市，他们的身份只是从农村贫困人口转变为了城市贫困人口，贫穷的状态没有发生改变。为了避免发生这种情况，中国的决策者们制定了相应措施，确保农民工能在城市的工业企业中找到工作，而这些企业也满足了全球日益增长的需求。

从某种意义上来说，城镇化是一种内生现象，因为在工业生产中，规模经济体量巨大，这也使得将工作集中在一个地方完成变得尤为重要。城镇化通过集聚效应优化了工业企业的物流系统。同时，城镇化也是劳动力在工业企业聚集的必然结果，能帮助劳动力解决就业问题。换言之，自1979年起，中国的城镇化经历了以下过程，即工业化先行，城镇化紧随其后，这意味着中国几乎没有遇到过城镇失业问题。在中国的发展史上，失业和贫困并不是工业化和城镇化的产物。

如果非要将中国从贫穷到繁荣崛起的过程总结成某个发展战略，我认为是两方面因素共同作用的结果，一是通过开放贸易拉动了全球的需求，二是按照正确的顺序进行了结构变革，从农村农业社会转变成了城市工业社会。中国居民收入的增长速度比历史上任何地方都快，同时社会各阶层的贫困率全面下降，这使得繁荣成果由全民共享。在中国收入最低的 40% 人群中，他们的收入增长速度比全国平均水平要快得多。

中国并不是唯一一个从贫穷的农业国家成功转变为繁荣的中等收入或富裕经济体的发展中国家（许多东亚和南亚发展中国家也实现了类似的转型）。全球贸易一体化程度进一步加深，全球价值链建立并完善，二者共同推动了这一繁荣景象。经济体之间相互关联，也称贸易依存，使得全球数十亿人成功摆脱了贫困。然而现在，人们正受到世界上某些国家经济民族主义和单边主义邪恶势力的威胁。

过去 70 年间，在关贸总协定和世贸组织等多边贸易体制下发展起来的以规则为基础的贸易体制暴露出一些治理框架方面的缺点。全球多边机构需要实施有效的改革，使机构更加现代化，跟上技术进步的步伐。正如一些成员国所暗示的那样，促使机构逐步解散的做法无异于不分良莠，全盘抛弃。不可否认的是，如果这些机构最终解散，那么世界上 8 亿多穷人中的大多数将是最终的输家。（董方源翻译）

原文：

Learning from China's War Against Poverty

Zaidi Sattar[*]

In 2015, the UN General Assembly adopted the Sustainable Develop-

* Zaidi Sattar, Chairman, Policy Research Institute of Bangladesh.

ment Goals (SDG) for eliminating poverty by 2030. It was an universal call to action to end poverty, protect the planet and ensure that all people enjoy peace and prosperity. The 17 goals committed under SDG 2030 were not only about eliminating poverty but these goals comprise a wholesome effort to improve the human condition around the globe, by devising effective policies to create wealth in an inclusive way, while sustainably harnessing the planet's abundant natural resources. So both creation and distribution of wealth is very much on the agenda.

With so much poverty and deprivation around, there can be little argument about the need to eradicate poverty around the globe, sooner rather than later. There is also no doubt that the road to end poverty is fraught with daunting challenges. So a 15-year road map makes a lot of sense, though questions remain about the feasibility of this time frame. How feasible is it? Historical and cross-country evidence offers some useful lessons for nations that are burdened with substantial poor population and with limited resources to fight poverty-in particular, the developing countries in Asia, Africa and Latin America. For them, no doubt the Chinese experience in reducing poverty could offer meaningful strategic guidance.

Though the emergence of COVID-19 pandemic adds a new dimension to the poverty challenge globally, China's 30-year experience with poverty reduction remains relevant for developing countries. China, the most populated country in the world, with 1.4 billion people, now has less than 10 million of its people regarded as extremely poor, i. e. living under $1.90 a day by the World Banks's criteria. In 2015, that worked out to 0.7 percent of the population compared to 53% in 1981. In three decades, China's development strategy was able to lift some 600 million people out of poverty. That could be considered one of the fastest rate of poverty reduction in history for such a vast population.

Globally, there has been marked progress on reducing poverty over the past decades. According to the most recent estimates, 9 percent of the world's population live on less than US $1.90 a day, down from nearly 36 percent in 1990. That would still leave some 780 million people in poverty today, more than half of China's population-an unacceptably high number, indicating that the benefits of economic growth have been shared unevenly across regions and countries. Countries in East Asia and the Pacific have been most successful in routing out poverty, followed by South Asia and Latin America; but Sub-Saharan Africa still remains stubbornly resistant to poverty reduction (Table 1).

Table 1   **Extreme poverty rates, by region, 1990 – 2015**

Region	Poverty rate (%) 1990	Poverty rate (%) 2015
East Asia and Pacific	61. 5	2. 3
South Asia	47. 3	12. 4
Latin America	14. 2	4. 1
Sub – Saharan Africa	54. 3	41. 1
World	35. 9	8. 6 *
China	53. 0 **	0. 7

Source of data: World Bank; (*) 2018, (**) 1981.

Poverty is indeed a curse regardless of where it is. The poor around the world live in squalor deprived of the basic necessities of life that the average person takes for granted-adequate food, housing, education, healthcare, and so on. In this 21st century of boundless technological advance the fact that 1 out of every 10 person in our world, i. e. nearly 800 million people, lives in poverty casts a long shadow on all the achievements human civilization has made over the past several centuries of progress. Key national and global challenges are standing in the way of progress and are keeping large pockets of people trapped in poverty. Slow growth, macroeconomic imbalances, escalating trade tensions, high levels of inequality in income and opportunities, climate change, and increasing fragility and conflict pose obstacles to further poverty reduction and inclusive growth.

It was therefore appropriate for the world community to finally realize that the time for action had come. But progress in eliminating global poverty has been uneven and falling short of what is needed for achieving the goal of zero extreme poverty by 2030. Even that seems not to be on track, according to recent forecasts. UN 2019 progress report on SDG finds that the number of people living in extreme poverty declined from 36% in 1990 to 8.6% in 2018, but the pace of poverty reduction is starting to decelerate as the world struggles to respond to entrenched deprivation, violent conflicts and vulnerabilities to natural disasters. Also, global hunger has been on the rise after a prolonged decline. These challenges have now been compounded by the COVID-19 pandemic that has disrupted economic activities globally, causing tremendous negative shock to output, employment and income in so many countries and regions. This could set the clock of poverty reduction a few steps backwards. With the COVID-19 pandemic upon us, which is a combined health and economic shock of unprecedented scale, it might now be practical to move the SDG target date to 2035.

So what are the key ingredients of a successful development strategy that is effective in eliminating poverty? Is there something developing countries can learn from the Chinese experience of rapid growth, job creation, and poverty reduction?

When China began its transition from a planned to a market-oriented economy in 1979, it was a poor, inward-looking country with a per capita income of US $182 and a trade dependence (trade-to-GDP) ratio of 11.2 percent. China's economic performance since then has been miraculous. Annual GDP growth averaged 10 percent over the 30-year period (1980 – 2010), and international trade averaged 16 percent per annum. China is now a upper middle-income country, and more than 600 million people have escaped poverty. Its trade dependence ratio has reached 65 percent, the highest among the world's large economies. In 2009 China overtook Japan as the world's second largest economy and replaced Germany as the world's largest exporter of merchandise. China is euphemistically called the world's "factory". What strategy of development brought this about?

It would be too simplistic to suggest there was one strategy that produced this outcome for China. But its switch towards greater openness and trade orientation, among other things, definitely played a pivotal role. In the 1960s and 1970s, a new paradigm of development emerged from East Asia and the Pacific—the paradigm of trade-led growth. The now famous East Asian Tiger economies showed the way to leverage the massive global market and grow faster. The vast global demand provided a deep, elastic market for their goods. China, in transition to more openness in 1979, went a step further. China was quick to recognize the criticality of two strategic sources of rapid growth—international trade and knowledge transfer. By opening up to trade in the international marketplace it wasable to exploit the vast global demand for its manufacturing output while importing knowledge that helped raise productive efficiency.

Just as important, China followed the right sequence for its industrialization: first, in contrast to the comparative-advantage-defying (CAD) import substitution strategy pursued by many developing countries, China's industrial expansion and exports was based on the country's vast army of cheap labor, a comparative-advantage-following (CAF) strategy. Next, it adopted greater technological sophistication by importing ideas, technology, and know-how from the rest of the world. China thus imported what the world knew and exported what the world wanted. World demand gave its industries the scale economies that the domestic market lacked.

A complementary strategy was in its pursuit of structural change that was inclusive in that job creation, industrialization and urbanization all went hand in hand. Historically, all countries in the world were poor and agrarian at the beginning of their modernization. For those few countries that successfully transformed from poverty to prosperity, they all converted from rural agrarian economies to urban industrialized economies. So did China but with a difference. When people move from rural areas to urban ones without jobs, they simply change from rural poor to urban poor. Poverty remains. To avoid this situation, Chinese policymakers made sure that the migrant labor force had jobs in urban industries which catered to rising world demand.

Urbanization is endogenous in some sense because in industrial production, the economies of scale are large, making concentration of work in one location important. While improving the logistical base of industries in terms of clustering or agglomeration, urbanization is the outcome of reinforcing the concentration of workforce and people around the agglomerated location of industries, which may help them to avoid unemployment. To some extent, under the transformation starting in 1979, China's urbanization followed this kind of process. Industrialization came first, and then urbanization, meaning that there were little urban unemployment issues in China. Unemployment and poverty were not the handmaiden of industrialization and urbanization in the Chinese development story.

If a singular development strategy could be attributed to China's rise from poverty to prosperity it was the combination of leveraging world demand through trade openness and executing the right sequence of structural transformation from rural-agrarian to urban-industrial societies. While incomes rose at rates faster than anywhere in history poverty declined all across the board reaching all strata of society, thus making prosperity very inclusive. The share of income of the bottom 40% grew much faster than the average.

China is not alone among developing countries that successfully transformed from poor agrarian economies to prosperous middle income or rich economies (e. g. many East Asian and South Asian developing economies fall in this category) . Greater global trade integration and the rise of Global Value Chains (GVCs) has been the common theme driving this prosperity. This interlinkage of economies—called trade dependence—that lifted billions of people across the globe out of poverty is now under threat from sinister forces of economic nationalism and unilateralism in some parts of the world.

While the rules-based trading system that evolved over the past 70 years under the multilateral trading regime of GATT-WTO has revealed some weaknesses in its governance framework, what the global multilateral institution needs is to be revamped with effective reforms to modernize the institution in keeping with the march of technological progress. To foster its gradual dissolution, as some members seem to hint at, would be like throwing the baby out with the bathwater. There is no denying that so many of the world's 800 million poor will be the ultimate losers if that prospect becomes real.

后　　记

　　《大变局下的博弈与合作》共收录 34 篇文章，其中外方前政要、专家学者贡献 28 篇、中方学者贡献 6 篇。

　　此论文集顺利出版，首先要感谢中国社会科学院高端智库首席专家、学部委员蔡昉教授，对此次约稿工作的悉心指导和大力支持。感谢每位为此书贡献论文的中外专家、学者，正是因为他们的勤勉敬业，才使得此书有了坚强的学识保障，让中外读者能够更加深刻地了解此次疫情带给世界的世纪变迁和人类为抗击疫情而付出的不懈努力。感谢中国社会科学出版社的大力支持，感谢中国社会科学院的毛悦、王文娥、杨莉、王晶、杜鹃、楼宇、徐璞玉、于海青、楼宇以及国际关系学院的董方源等翻译人员，以及感谢智库秘书处工作人员叶莹菲、任志娇、赫雅菲、李立婷在对外联络、书稿整理等方面所做的工作。

　　正是由于上述诸位的共同努力，保证本书的及时付梓与应有的专业水准。特此鸣谢！

Afterword

Game and Cooperation under Profound Changes includes a total of 34 articles, twenty-eight by former foreign dignitaries, experts and scholars, and six by Chinese scholars.

Regarding the successful publication of the symposiums, first of all, I would like to thank Professor Cai Fang, Chief Expert of the National High-end Think Tank at the and Secretary-General of the CASS Presidium of Academic Divisions, for his careful guidance on and strong support for the call for contributions. I would also express my gratitude to every Chinese and foreign experts and scholars for their contributions. It is their dedication that greatly enriches the book so that readers at home and abroad can have a deeper understanding of the historic changes brought by the pandemic and the unremitting efforts to fight the coronavirus. I am extremely grateful to the China Social Sciences Press for its vigorous support, to Mao Yue, Wang Wen'e, Yang Li, Wang Jing, Du Juan, Lou Yu, Xu Puyu, Yu Haiqing of the Chinese Academy of Social Sciences and Dong Fangyuan of the University of International Relations for their translation work, and to Ye Yingfei, Ren Zhijiao, He Yafei, and Li Liting who work in the think tank secretariat for their external liaison and arrangement of contributions.

It is the joint efforts of you all that guarantee the timely publication and high quality of the book. Special thanks to you all!